A CASE OF CULTURE

HOW CULTURAL BROKERS BRIDGE DIVIDES IN HEALTHCARE

Happy reading!

SNIGDHA NANDIPATI

Snigdha Nandipati

NEW DEGREE PRESS

A CASE OF CULTURE
How Cultural Brokers Bridge Divides in Healthcare

ISBN   978-1-63730-835-6   *Paperback*
         978-1-63730-899-8   *Kindle Ebook*
         978-1-63730-952-0   *Ebook*

"No one culture has ever developed all human potentialities; it has always selected certain capacities, mental and emotional and moral, and stifled others. Each culture is a system of values which may well complement the values in another."

—RUTH BENEDICT

Om Namo Narayanaya Namaha
To Amma, for showing me how beautiful our culture is.
To Daddy, for inspiring me to reach for the stars.
And to Sujan, for being my anchor of
support through thick and thin.
This book is for you.

TABLE OF CONTENTS

INTRODUCTION

I couldn't breathe. My nose was so stuffed with boogers and snot that the only way I could breathe was to keep my mouth open and pant like a dog. The hairs on my seven-year-old arms stood up, forming small goosebumps all over.

"*Amma,*" I wheezily tried to shout. No response. "*Ammaaaaa!*"

I lay shivering under my pink flower-printed blankie for what felt like hours, hoping that someone would come to my rescue. At long last, I heard the thump of footsteps and the jingle of Amma's bangles as she walked toward my room.

"*Vaana lo thadavaddhani cheppana?* Didn't I warn you about playing in the rain?" Amma chided me. "Now the rain got you wet and gave you *jalubu* (common cold)."

I nodded, my teeth chattering from the cold.

"*Undu, vedi vedi ga miriyala paalu theeskostha.* I will bring some warm pepper milk for you." She left the room toward the kitchen to make the *miriyala paalu.*

After some minutes, Amma returned with a small steel glass in her hands and sat next to me on my twin-sized bed. I peered into the glass and found a pale brown-colored liquid with small black specks floating in it.

My nose scrunched up in disgust. "*Naaku odhu!* I don't want it!" I wailed.

"If you want to feel better, you have to drink it," Amma said.

According to Amma, *miriyala paalu,* like ripe mango and dried coconut and *rasam* (a spicy watery tomato soup popular in South India), was a "hot" food that would increase my body heat and cure my cold. Bananas and fennel seeds and *perugu* (plain curd), on the other hand, were "cold" foods that would reduce body heat and cure a fever or sore throat. I didn't know much about the Ayurvedic principles behind these practices. All I knew was that I would never play in the rain again if it meant I would have to drink *miriyala paalu.*

I sat silently next to Amma, considering my options. I could either brave the *miriyala paalu* concoction, or I could stay here shivering under my blankets. After some deliberation, I conceded.

"Only if I get to watch *Hanuman* after," I countered. I had seen this cartoon movie at least fifty times already, yet it remained my favorite. I stretched out my tiny hand and held the small steel glass. The warmth of the glass in my hands felt amazing. I put it to my lips and took a sip. It tasted exactly as I imagined it would. It was spicy and warm and burned my throat as I swallowed it. A small piece of black pepper ball got caught in my throat and I started gagging.

"Amma!" I wailed. "I don't want to drink it anymore!"

"Please, *thalli. Naa kosam.* For me."

I pinched my nose and gulped down the rest.

* * *

My family's medicine cabinet was never stocked with Tylenol or Dayquil like in other homes. Instead, jars of turmeric, dried basil leaves, black pepper balls, ginger powder, *kasturi* pills, and other kitchen ingredients lined the shelves of our bathroom. This is the approach to health that my family has preserved for generations. In my family where tradition and culture are kept alive through a myriad of ways, Ayurveda had also worked itself into our daily practices. My family trusts our turmeric more than any Tylenol to keep us healthy because it is what we know best. It is our *familiar.*

Consequently, my brother and I grew up with an unfamiliarity of most over-the-counter medications. I had only taken Tylenol around ten times my entire life, the majority of those times having taken place in the last couple of years after I moved out of the house.

According to a 2014 study by pharmacologist Martins Ekor, it has been estimated that up to 80 percent of the world's population in the Global South relies on herbal remedies as their primary source of healthcare and views traditional healing practices as an important part of their culture. When these families emigrate from the Global South to other countries, they carry their culture with them, herbal remedies and all. In my family, our healing traditions were very much a part of our culture and practices. My family didn't see value in using medication for something we could heal using ingredients we already had at home. They had been passed down to us across generations through the experiences and wisdom of our ancestors. If our methods worked for our grandparents, great-grandparents, and great-great-grandparents, why wouldn't they work for us?

Not to mention, our traditional methods of healing were much more affordable and easier to obtain compared to medications from the pharmacy. We didn't have to drive to the nearest CVS in search of Neosporin or Tums that would expire in a year or two anyway. We had our own medicines right here in our kitchen: a mixture of *pasupu* (turmeric) and *kobbari noona* (coconut oil) in place of Neosporin, and *kasturi* pills (small black balls made of a concoction of dried spices and herbs) in place of Tums.

When the time came for me to leave for college, Amma packed my suitcases with many small glass jars and Ziplocs filled with turmeric, ginger powder, *kasturi* pills, basil leaves, and all the other ingredients that would help protect me against the dreaded dorm room germs. For the first two years of college, I somehow managed to escape the need for these items, but my luck ran short in my third year.

I came down with the flu in mid-March, the day before my a cappella group's biggest concert of the year. *How wonderful.* Not only did I have chills and a sore throat, but I also lost my voice. I had never experienced this before, so I was particularly horrified when I opened my mouth to speak and nothing but a small croak escaped. How in the world would I recover in time to sing my solo tomorrow?

For the first time, I opened the jar of ginger powder that Amma had packed in my suitcase. It was tightly sealed shut from the years of being left unopened in the back of my dorm room dresser. I made myself a concoction of ginger tea with honey to drink at bedtime with the hope that I would feel better in the morning.

I woke up the next morning feeling just as crappy as I did the day before. The good news was that my voice had returned. The bad news was that I had a 101-degree fever and was too fatigued to even sit up, let alone perform on stage for three hours. Not to mention, I didn't think I would be able to hit any of the high notes in my "Hallelujah" solo. I made myself some more ginger tea as I deliberated. Should I call the musical director and let her know I couldn't make it? Or should I just suck it up and do my best, even if I end up sounding like a dying hyena on stage for my last concert ever? I was frozen with indecision.

Taylor, my roommate, saw me sitting in my bed with my cup of tea, clutching my head.

"Isn't your concert tonight?" she asked.

"Yeah," I groaned. "I don't want to miss it, but I may not have a choice."

"You look terrible. Did you take Tylenol?"

I shook my head no.

"Girl. How are you gonna be a doctor and pre-scribe medications to others if you won't even take them yourself?"

Taylor had a point. I wasn't comfortable with taking over-the-counter medicines because it was something I never grew up doing, but I had already tried my home remedies the night before and they were unsuccessful. Besides the return of my voice, I wasn't feeling much better. I was in a race against time to get well before my concert that evening.

She handed me a Tylenol and told me to get some sleep. The least I could do was try. If it worked, great. Otherwise, I'd be in the same boat as I was now. I gingerly took it, swallowed it down forcefully with some water, and got back under my blanket.

Several hours later, my alarm rang. I woke up from my nap, and to my surprise, my head was no longer pounding. I was able to stand up without keeling over, and my fever had mostly subsided. I wondered how it was possible that a single pill was enough to do the job. Maybe it was just some really strong Tylenol. Or maybe it was that my body had no tolerance to Tylenol because I never grew up taking it. Or maybe, just maybe, my ginger tea and extra hours of sleep were starting to kick in.

I rushed to get ready and headed to the concert hall in my heels and black gown. Though I still wasn't feeling my best, I was able to sing my "Hallelujah" solo *and* hit all the high notes, which was much more than I could have hoped for that morning.

To this day, I can't quite articulate why I hesitate to use medication. Logically, I know that these medications have passed many checkpoints in clinical trials, but for some reason I still instinctively reach for the ginger powder before the Tylenol. Even though I was born and raised here in the United States, my cultural upbringing has pulled me toward the health attitudes and beliefs I hold today.

This episode was an important step for me in realizing that unless I made peace with my own conflicting views of medicine and healing, I could not expect my future patients to do so either. Yet, at the same time, I realized this process of learning to balance my own cultural beliefs with my health needs has equipped me to be a more effective advocate to those patients who face similar dilemmas.

* * *

The United States is a country of ever-increasing diversity. According to the 2000 US Census Bureau, there were around seventy million people from nineteen non-European ethnic and cultural groups living in the US. With each of these groups comes a unique set of cultural beliefs about health and illness. Some swear by using antibiotics for every condition, while others won't even touch medication unless it is all natural. Some believe that illness is due to an imbalance of good and bad energies, while others believe that illness is caused by evil-eye or dark spirits. Some prefer family members or elders take care of the individual's health-related matters, while others forbid disclosing anything about one's personal health to even the closest of family.

As you can imagine, it is close to impossible for people from every one of these diverse cultural groups to find a physician that knows and understands the cultural beliefs they hold about health and illness. Similarly, it is close to impossible that a physician is competent and knowledgeable about the cultural beliefs of every single patient they see.

At the end of the day, what patients want is to be listened to and understood by their physicians. Likewise, what physicians want is to help empower their patients toward taking ownership of their health in the way that best fits their needs and goals. But when there exists a discrepancy in language and literacy, distrust of the medical system, unfamiliarity with Western medical practices, differences in health beliefs, varying emotional states of mind, and many other barriers to communication, it can be extremely difficult for the patient to open up with their doctor. To top it off, our physicians work in a healthcare system that burns them out, that prioritizes quantity over quality, and that gives them ten to fifteen minutes per patient max (Linzer, 2015). With all of this on the plate, the patient's hope of being understood threatens to become just that...a lost hope.

A very special group of people ensures that patients can receive the culturally concordant care they need: cultural brokers. According to the Jezewski model, cultural brokering is defined as "the act of bridging, linking, or mediating between groups or persons of different cultural backgrounds for the purpose of reducing conflict or producing change." The practice of cultural brokering is actually quite ancient, dating back thousands of years to the first recorded encounters between groups of different cultures. From encounters between ancient Macedonians and Persians in the third century BCE, to those between Anglo-Europeans and Native Americans in the eighteenth century, cultural brokers were crucial to bridging divides across these cultures in order to enact change and mediate conflict.

The term "broker" is used in many industries and contexts to refer to the middleman who facilitates the flow of information between two parties. For example, brokers are an important part of the financial and real estate industries because their knowledge of both buyers and sellers allows them to serve as an effective means of communication. The buyer may not understand all the jargon and technical terms that a seller uses, or perhaps the buyer is unable to make a financial negotiation because he lacks the necessary knowledge. In such cases, the broker steps in to help the buyer make sense of the various industry rules and regulations, explaining them in layman's terms. By helping ease communication and build trust between the buyer and seller, the broker helps to establish a meaningful relationship between the two parties.

In a similar vein, cultural brokers facilitate between the culture of the (often) foreign-born patient, the culture of the host country where the patient seeks care, and the culture of the healthcare system itself. Sometimes the patient may not agree with what the doctor suggests because it is at odds with their cultural beliefs. Other times, the patient may be overwhelmed by the many moving parts of a foreign healthcare system and needs help with navigating it. In such situations, the cultural broker steps in to ease these interactions between patient and provider, mitigating any misunderstandings that may arise in the process. This process of cultural brokering in the healthcare system can be carried out by anyone who has an understanding of both cultures. This might be an interpreter, a priest, a patient advocate, a family member, and sometimes even the doctor themselves.

As every child of immigrants knows (myself included), playing broker becomes second nature as we help our families navigate the challenges of living two cultures at once. But it wasn't until I entered my current professional role as a patient advocate that I came to realize exactly how irreplaceable our cultural upbringing and experiences are in the healthcare setting. I understood diabetic Mr. M's cultural attachment to rice. I encouraged turmeric-reliant Ms. B to get vaccinated against COVID-19. I saw first-hand the amalgamation of cultural, linguistic, and spiritual barriers that exacerbated the health conditions of our immigrant patients, and I realized how my dual-identity upbringing had equipped me to help our patients overcome these barriers.

Some people believe that having a cultural broker, having this extra third wheel, gets in the way of the sacred patient-doctor relationship, but I disagree. I believe that having a cultural broker *enhances* the patient-doctor relationship. The cultural broker encourages the patient to be more open and communicative with their doctor, assuring them that their doctor can and will help them achieve their health goals. Likewise, the cultural broker educates the doctor about the cultural beliefs of the patient that may conflict with the care being provided. Cultural brokers are important for helping both patients and doctors navigate their care accordingly. Just as the doctor's goal is to treat their patient so well that the doctor is no longer needed, the broker's goal is to facilitate such a trusting and open patient-doctor relationship so that the broker is no longer needed.

There is an ever-increasing plethora of data and research on the importance of culture and diversity in providing healthcare, but it is the stories of these middlemen that get lost in the fray. So, I wrote this book about us, the oft-forgotten cultural brokers. I wrote this anthology of personal narratives, positive experiences, and cautionary tales with the hope of bringing to light the countless efforts of cultural brokers in healthcare. Whether it's the son who encourages his Italian father to open up to his doctor about his medication noncompliance, the Mongolian interpreter who assures her patient that HIPAA would protect her personal health information (unlike in her home country), the Internal Medicine intern who encourages his patient to open up about her heavy period (a culturally stigmatized topic) with her doctor, or the ICU hospitalist who calls her patient "Aunty" to help her feel more at home in this strange environment and new country, each of the stories in this book shares the importance of the cultural broker in building, facilitating, and enhancing the patient-doctor relationship.

CHAPTER 1

THE WELL FROG

"A well-frog cannot imagine the ocean, nor can a summer insect conceive of ice. How then can a scholar understand the Tao? He is restricted by his own learning."

— BENJAMIN HOFF

It was a blistery snowy night in a small town in upstate New York, and the icy roads were almost entirely empty. Around ten o'clock that night, a middle-aged Vietnamese couple rushed to the local hospital's emergency room with their eight-year-old son. Their son had been suffering from a high fever for almost five days now. He would not stop coughing, his nose was constantly running, and he complained of severe backaches.

The son was assigned to a room to wait in with his parents. A nurse walked in and began to collect his vitals. 103-degree temperature—high fever. 120/70 mm Hg—normal blood pressure. 90 bpm—strong rhythmic and regular pulse. 22 breaths per minute—slight heaviness with breathing, but otherwise normal rate.

The doctor entered the room to perform the examination. "Say aaaah." He looked inside the boy's mouth with a scope, holding his tongue down with a wooden tongue depressor. The back of his throat was colored a violent red, and his tonsils were so inflamed and swollen that they blocked much of his airway. This was a classic sign of bacterial tonsillitis and was something that could be easily treated with a few days of amoxicillin (an antibiotic).

Just to confirm his suspected diagnosis, the doctor lifted the boy's patient gown to listen to his lung sounds. When he did, he was met with a strange sight. The boy's back was covered with large black and blue marks that ran down the length of his torso in straight vertical lines. The boy winced as the doctor gently touched the bruises.

When there is a case of trauma that leaves behind scars in a particular pattern or formation, it is usually assumed these injuries are intentionally inflicted upon the individual. This boy's bruises decorated his back in a striking black and blue zebra-stripe pattern, as if he were whipped or beaten with a long rigid board. Naturally, the doctor figured this was a case of child abuse. Child Protective Services was summoned, and the boy was taken away from his parents.

It wasn't until many hours later that the parents were able to get the help of a Vietnamese interpreter. Though the population in this area of upstate New York was largely Caucasian and homogenous, for some reason or another, there was a moderately large Vietnamese community that had settled there. This made it easier for the parents to get the help they needed and to explain to the medical team that this was not a case of abuse.

Rather, this was an instance of *cao gio* (coining), a traditional healing method that is commonly used in Southeast Asia to rid the body of its "extra heat" and "negative energy." Each country has its own name for the practice of coining. In Vietnam, coining is called *cao gio*, which means "to scratch out the wind." In China, it is called *gua sha*, which means "scraping sand." Cambodians call it *kos kyal*, Indonesians call it *kerik*, and Laotians call it *khoud lam* (Darsha, 2020).

To perform coining, the skin is first covered in an herbal oil, camphor balm, or other lubricant. Then, the edge of a coin or other small hard object is pressed and rubbed against the skin in a linear fashion. This process is repeated until red lines of bruising appear, which is taken as a sign of the "extra heat" leaving the body. The larger and more numerous the red lines, the greater the release of heat and the more successful the coining process (Tan, 2011).

Even though the boy's doctor was right to infer these injuries were intentionally inflicted upon the boy, as was demonstrated by the patterned bruising, there are instances in which injuries are inflicted without the intent to do harm. This was one such exception. Many folk remedies and cultural methods of healing (including coining, cupping, and moxibustion) inflict wounds on the skin that can be easily mistaken for abuse by those who are not familiar with these cultural practices.

The US Census Bureau estimates that almost 20 percent of the US population will be foreign-born by the year 2060 (Colby, 2015). And yet, the scientific literature shows little about the different healing methods, perceptions of illness, and beliefs around health that these different cultures carry. Hearing this boy's story led me to realize one thing: this is why cultural brokers matter. Because the Vietnamese interpreter was able to serve as a cultural broker and explain the reason behind this bruising pattern to the medical team, the hospital realized these parents were wrongly accused of abuse. The boy was reunited with his family and a complicated legal situation was avoided. The cultural broker was vital to ensuring proper care and maintaining trust.

* * *

Years ago, I began reading the works of Swami Vivekananda. His wisdom was profound, and I was not yet at the age or maturity to understand it all. But one story he did share, a story he would go on to narrate at his notable speech at the 1893 Parliament of the World's Religions, was the first thing that came to my mind when I learned about the case of this Vietnamese boy. Swami Vivekananda told a story of a frog that lived in a well, that was born and brought up there and spent its entire life believing its small well to be the entire world. One day, another frog came and fell into the well.

"Where are you from?" the first frog asked.

"I am from the sea," the second frog responded.

"The sea! How big is that? Is it as big as my well?" and he took a leap from one side of the well to the other.

"My friend," said the frog of the sea, "how can you compare the sea with your little well?"

Then the frog took another leap and asked, "Is your sea so big?"

The frog of the sea exclaimed, "What nonsense you speak, to compare the sea with your well!"

"Well, then," said the frog of the well, "nothing can be bigger than my well; there can be nothing bigger than this; this fellow is a liar, so turn him out."

It was as Swami Vivekananda explained, and as Benjamin Hoff alluded to in his quote at the beginning of this chapter: "I am sitting in my own well and thinking that the whole world is my little well." It is our own experiences that restrict us from considering the possibility that there are experiences and customs and practices and cultures beyond our own that are equally valid. As Hoff says, "[We are] restricted by [our] own learning."

These misunderstandings, these biases and preconceived notions, are not isolated to any one culture. They happen more frequently than we might think. And more often than not, there's a grim ending to the story. Every culture has its own set of beliefs, and as a result, its own set of misunderstandings when it comes into contact with another culture.

In fact, just the other week as I was discharging the last patient in our COVID vaccine clinic, I received a notification in my email inbox. "Hindu Mom Needs Help," the subject line read. It was an email from my volunteer coordinator. She and I volunteer together for a national grassroots organization that works to improve the understanding of Hinduism and Dharmic culture in North America. I opened the email and began to read.

"A Hindu mom called me last week with a pitiful tale. Her seven-year-old daughter was taken away by the city's Department of Human Services under 'child abuse' because the department did not understand Hindu cultural practices."

The laptop almost slipped from my limp hands. I continued to read.

I learned the mother had given her daughter an *abhyanga snana*. *Abhyanga snana* is a customary health practice in Hindu culture in which a warm fragrant herb-infused oil is massaged into the body from head to toe before bathing or showering. It is believed in Ayurveda that the *abhyanga snana* is important for improving strength, health, and longevity.

The daughter brought up her *abhyanga snana* in conversation with her friends at school, only she must have provided a crude English translation for *abhyanga snana* as "oil bath." Soon enough, the news of her oil bath made its way to her teachers, who became extremely concerned that this was a situation of abuse in which her mother was *literally* dunking her in a bath of oil. A series of miscommunications and heightened emotions led the school to call the Department of Human Services to "rescue" the daughter from her "abusive" mother. The daughter was transferred to foster care, where she had been staying for over a month. The mother, who has been forced to live in a hotel, has only been allowed to see her daughter with an appointment.

My stomach turned. What if I were in that daughter's place? Or in that mother's place? To think a family could be torn apart at a moment's notice, simply because no one bothered to understand what actually took place or to learn what this cultural practice was.

What made this situation particularly tragic and unacceptable was the school's response to the situation.

Instead of performing their own investigation before jumping to conclusions, the school simply handed off the responsibility of cross-cultural brokership to the daughter, even when she wasn't prepared to do so. She was too young to fulfill the expectations the school had placed upon her.

In order to effectively mediate between different cultural beliefs, a cultural broker must have these three qualities, according to the National Center for Cultural Competence at Georgetown University:

1. awareness
2. knowledge
3. skills

First, the cultural broker must have awareness of their own cultural identity and how it differs from the broader cultural identity at large. According to Piaget's Stages of Psychosocial Development, children from ages two to seven are in the pre-operational stage, as was the daughter in this case. In this stage, her intelligence and thought processes are *egocentric*. This means she naturally assumes what she knows and sees is what everyone else around her knows and sees. She knows what an *oil bath* is, so surely others must know as well. She is unable to understand that other people have different bases of knowledge upon which they build their awareness, which might affect how they imagine an *oil bath*. Importantly, she struggles to think outside of her own perspective.

Next, a good cultural broker has knowledge of both cultures they mediate between. They have a thorough understanding of the values, beliefs, and practices that are associated with their cultural group, as well as the viewpoints and perspectives the broader Western or "host" culture carries. Importantly, they have knowledge and intuition of how these two cultures differ and what misunderstandings might arise as a result of their contact. While the daughter grew up as the child of two cultures, Indian and American, she was not yet at the age where she could differentiate and mediate between these two cultures. She herself was still learning about how the traditions her family practiced were different from those of her friends' families. As such, she was in no position to predict and respond to resulting misunderstandings.

Finally, a good cultural broker has the necessary skills to communicate ideas across cultures, which often requires knowledge and fluency in multiple languages. Importantly, they are able to manage misunderstandings and mediate conflict should they arise. The daughter was at a stage where she was still developing her language and communication skills, in two starkly different languages and cultural contexts no less. Though she was semantically correct to translate *abhyanga snana* into English as *oil bath*, she was unable to recognize that the term *oil bath* could be interpreted with a very different meaning than what she intended.

Her difficulties with these components of cross-cultural communication ultimately prevented her from serving as an effective cultural broker. Out of desperation, the mother reached out to our Hindu volunteer organization to help her with this case. With the help of our social work team, we were able to support the mother in proving to the Child Protective Services (CPS) that this was a case of cross-cultural misunderstanding and not child abuse.

Despite this victory, I couldn't help but think to myself: Why did the mother have to be the one to reach out for these services from us, when it was the negligence of the school and the cultural insensitivity of CPS that led to the unnecessary separation of this family?

If CPS took the liberty to accept false claims made by the school in alleging that this was a case of abuse, then it should have been their responsibility to check their facts before taking action. It was foolish of the school to expect a seven-year-old girl to take on this role, and it was unfair of CPS to require the mother to reach out for the assistance that should have been provided by CPS in the first place. It was CPS's duty to reach out to us or any other cultural broker well-versed in Hindu practices to fact check the situation before reporting abuse and taking custody of the child.

Now, the Vietnamese parents and Hindu mother were fortunate to be able to reach out for cultural brokering support, even though the onus should not have been on either of them to do so. Perhaps they were successful because of the respective cultural communities in which they lived. Perhaps the contacts within their communities were knowledgeable about both the culture's practices and the healthcare and legal systems, allowing them to act as a bridge. But what happens when this sort of misunderstanding occurs in a culture that is dying, in a culture where few individuals are capable of bridging these two starkly different cultural systems? What are the consequences of not having someone available to take on the role of a cultural broker?

* * *

Some months ago, I was reading a case study in a Health Literacy textbook in which a young woman had taken her elderly Navajo grandfather to a local internal medicine clinic in a small Arizona town (Health Literacy, 2004). He had an infection on his right leg that was growing larger and larger as the days passed. Unable to bear the pain of his leg and the berating of his granddaughter, he agreed to go to the clinic with her.

During the appointment, the doctor took a look at the infection. It was already pretty severe, and it could have led to the grandfather losing his leg had he waited any longer to come in.

"You came to us at the right time. You need to take this medication if you want to treat this infection. Otherwise, it can get a lot worse," the doctor said.

The grandfather, who did not know English, couldn't understand a word the doctor was telling him. The granddaughter offered to serve as an interpreter for her grandfather, but unfortunately her knowledge of medical terminology in Navajo was limited. As she attempted to convey to her grandfather what the doctor was trying to say, she struggled to translate the word "infection" into Navajo.

Now, language is possibly the most complex and extensive representation of a group's culture. But when a culture lacks a certain concept or uses different means to explain a concept, there is often no direct translation available to explain said concept. For example, the Hmong culture has no direct word-to-word translation for "chemotherapy" because they have no concept of cancer as a disease. In fact, there is no word for cancer either. The word that they use for cancer translates to "death." Cancer is viewed as a fatalistic condition, in which cancer marks one's unchangeable destiny of death. So, in order to translate "chemotherapy," one would have to resort to a several-pages-long explanation of what cancer is, what chemotherapy treatment does to the body, and what the patient might experience as a result of receiving chemotherapy (Baisch, 2008).

This undoubtedly requires much knowledge of both the culture of the patient and the culture of the Western healthcare system, as well as experience with working within both of these starkly different cultural groups. Inexperience or lack of knowledge of either culture can lead to dire consequences. One inexperienced interpreter attempted to explain the idea of "radiation treatment" to a Hmong patient, who had no concept of cancer as a disease, let alone of radiation as a treatment. "We're going to put a fire in you," the interpreter explained poorly. Needless to say, the patient was horrified and refused treatment entirely (Morse, 2003).

This was exactly what happened with the Navajo grandfather. In the Navajo culture, there is no concept of "infection," since disease is believed to be a result of anything from improper conduction of rituals to accidental contact with *chindis* (evil ghosts), to breaking taboos set in place by the Holy People. There is no concept of bacteria or microorganisms that can enter a wound and release toxins and incite an immune system response. The closest Navajo interpretation of infection is "contamination," or the idea that inappropriate contact with animals, natural phenomena, or witches can cause illness (Csordas, 1989).

The granddaughter struggled to explain the concept of "infection" to her grandfather, who sat there confused about what was going on. The doctor asked one of the nurses to help with interpretation. Though the nurse was well-versed with the patient's case and understood the basis of his bacterial infection, she too was unsuccessful in conveying this concept into the patient's own language.

The grandfather grew frustrated from the confusion and lack of clarity. He just wanted to get out of there and find someone who actually knew what was going on and could explain it to him properly. So, he did what most patients do when they don't understand what the doctor is saying. He nodded as if to say "okay," pretending to understand what was going on.

Turning to the nurse, the grandfather told her in the Navajo language that he planned to have a traditional ritual performed for him in the next few days in order to heal the infection. He wanted to let the doctor know. The nurse translated this to the doctor, who simply nodded and once more emphasized the importance of taking medications to heal the infection, not once acknowledging the healing ceremony the patient was hoping to do. The frustrated grandfather, who still didn't understand what was wrong with his leg or why these medications were so important, just insisted that he understood and that he wanted to seek the help of a healer. With that, the doctor handed the patient a prescription for antibiotics and left the room.

The next day, the frustrated grandfather sought the help of a *hatali*. A *hatali* is a Navajo medicine man who is called upon to perform healing ceremonies and to act as a bridge to transfer power from the Holy People to the patient. Each *hatali* begins as an apprentice, assisting their teacher and assembling *jish* (medicine bundles) for ceremonies, until they are deemed fit to practice independently. Often times, the songs and chants performed during healing ceremonies are passed down from generation to generation within families. However, just as Western medicine has doctors that spend the majority of their life practicing in a particular specialty, Navajo *hatalii* similarly spend much of their lifetime learning and perfecting only a few songs and chants. These chants require much time, skill, and experience to learn and perfect. If these chants are not uttered perfectly, the Holy People can become angry, and the patient can suffer severe consequences as a result (Davies, 2002).

The *hatali* did his best to heal the grandfather, using the nine-day long Night Way healing ceremony. Each day, the grandfather was cleansed using a number of different exercises such as sand painting and sweat baths in order to attract the power of the Holy People and repel the evil *chindis* (Strom, 2021). But unfortunately, his infection continued to grow during these nine days.

While the granddaughter and the nurse were well-versed in Western medical practices but poor in the Navajo language, the *hatali* was the opposite. He was incredibly knowledgeable about the spiritual and cultural aspects of the grandfather's health and was fluent in Navajo. But when it came to understanding Western medical practices and how they might work to treat the grandfather, the *hatali* was close to illiterate. The granddaughter took her grandfather back to the clinic for treatment, but the infection had spread so rapidly that the entire leg had to be amputated. The doctor deemed it to be a result of "medication noncompliance."

Tragedies like these can only be prevented when those involved are able to transcend the "well-frog" mentality and acknowledge other world views as equally valid. But when that is not feasible (which is more often than not), the cultural broker works to bring out the best of both worlds to treat the patient and prevent misunderstandings like these from occurring. A good cultural broker is one that knows the practices of both Western medicine and cultural healing. But as we've seen, it's not so easy to come by those who are entirely knowledgeable or understanding of these two distinct worlds. As forces of Westernization continue to uproot and obliterate cultural practices, it will only become harder to find individuals who will be able to serve as necessary cultural brokers.

CHAPTER 2

A SHORE OF FAMILIARITY

"If you talk to a man in a language he understands, that goes to his head. If you talk to him in his own language, that goes to his heart."

— NELSON MANDELA

It was about three o'clock on an early August Thursday, and the late afternoon sun began to shine through the large windows of our clinic's waiting room. An elderly Punjabi Sikh man (let's call him Mr. Singh) walked up to the clinic doors to check in for his appointment. He was a new patient of ours who was stuck here in the US due to COVID-19 travel restrictions that prevented him from returning to New Delhi. He had been having stomach pain as of late but had no primary care doctor in San Francisco that could see him, nor did he have any health insurance that would allow him to access a primary care doctor. His friend, who was also a patient of ours, had told him about how our clinic offers primary care for free to those who have no insurance.

As Mr. Singh stood outside our clinic doors, the receptionist began to screen him for COVID exposure, asking him various questions through the intercom.

- "Have you had any fever, sore throat, or cough in the last two weeks?"
- "Have you had any loss of taste or smell recently?"
- "Have you had contact with anyone who has tested positive for COVID-19?"
- "Have you traveled outside the Bay Area in the last two weeks?"

He paused after each question with a blank expression on his face, then shook his head no. The receptionist let him in.

Mr. Singh stepped into the clinic waiting room with a slight limp in his gait. He was well dressed in a matching navy shirt and turban, with his navy-blue mask tucked neatly underneath where it reached his ears. His ears were fully covered by the turban, and his beard was largely covered by his cloth mask (with the exception of a few salt-and-pepper hairs that peeked out from underneath his mask). The corners of his eyes were lined with crow's feet, the mark of a normally jolly man, but today his eyes carried something else: fear.

Mr. Singh gingerly sat down in one of the freshly wiped-down black leather chairs of the waiting room, at a far enough distance from the other patient who was also sitting in the waiting room. I caught his eye from behind the front desk, and his expression seemed to soften a bit. "A fellow Indian," he must have thought. He folded his hands together in a *namaste* greeting, and I did the same in return.

The receptionist then approached him with a pale blue surgical mask in hand.

"Hi Mr. Singh! Could you please wear this surgical mask? We require that everyone wear a surgical mask in place of a cloth mask."

Mr. Singh took the mask from the receptionist and looked at it for a second. His eyes grew big, and he glanced over at me with panic. "Please...bring her?" He pointed toward me, the brown Indian girl. "*Vo samajhayegi.* She will understand." The receptionist motioned for me to come over and help, so I stepped out from behind the front desk and approached Mr. Singh.

"*Sat sri akal*," I greeted him.

Unfortunately, that was the extent of my knowledge of Punjabi, but he didn't seem to care. Something else was bothering him. He looked down at the mask with a panicked expression, and then looked back up at me. And that's when it dawned on me.

In the Sikh faith, one's hair is regarded as a gift of God's creation and therefore is something that should not be tampered with. As such, Sikhs keep their hair long (called *kesh*) and refrain from cutting it, both as a way to demonstrate appreciation for God's gift and to keep their focus off their appearance. Sikh men wear a turban or other form of head covering (e.g., *patka, parna,* or *dumalla* for boys and young men) when in public to keep their *kesh* neat, to show respect by keeping their heads covered, and to demonstrate equality among the faith's followers. For Sikh men, the turban is a core part of their culture and identity (Singh, 2021).

Mr. Singh's turban covered not only his hair but also both of his ears, as well as the ear straps of his cloth mask.

He must have worn his cloth mask at home before tying his turban on top to secure it. In order for him to wear the surgical mask given to him by the receptionist, he would have to fit the ear loops around his ears and, in the process, remove (or at least uncomfortably adjust) his turban in the middle of the waiting room, in front of everyone. No wonder he was panicked.

But on the other hand, it was clinic policy that every individual wear a surgical mask due to risk of COVID transmission, Mr. Singh included. How could we adhere to our clinic policy while simultaneously preserving the respect and dignity of our patient?

A strange memory came to mind. For the past several months, my mother had been watching various Hindi serials, in which the characters have been wearing face masks due to COVID. I remember one particular character who wore a turban, and his cloth mask was unlike what I had typically seen. Instead of ear loops, his mask had one long continuous band of cloth that looped around the back of his turban and kept his mask snugly tied to his face.

"This could work," I thought.

I took the surgical mask from the receptionist and grabbed a rubber band from inside one of our front desk drawers. We took some scissors, snipped the rubber band to create a long rubber string, then tied the ends of the string to either ear loop on the surgical mask to create a makeshift mask strap. Mr. Singh took the rubber band mask contraption and slipped the mask on over his turban and cloth mask, with the rubber band pressed snugly against the back of his turban. For a hastily tied rubber band, the fit was surprisingly good. He pulled down his hidden cloth mask slightly so that he could cover his beard fully as well. Mr. Singh's crow's feet crinkled, and the fear in his eyes seemed to disappear.

I am not Punjabi Sikh, nor have I ever experienced what it is like to wear a turban, but I did grow up around other Punjabi uncles in my community (and luckily was able to remember that particular episode of my mother's Hindi serial). I understood how important the turban was to Mr. Singh and how it might pose a challenge for him to adhere to the expectations that we had placed upon him (in other words, wearing this face mask).

We very well could have sought permission to adjust the protocol for this patient, but that would have invited many questions about his lack of surgical mask from the other staff and doctors who would interact with him later on during the visit. He already appeared nervous and uncomfortable, and to draw any more attention to how he wasn't fitting into our standards of care was unnecessary and undesirable. As basic as it was, our rubber band contraption seemed to be the best way to help Mr. Singh feel most integrated and welcomed while simultaneously respecting his cultural practices and beliefs.

Having a Punjabi Sikh on our staff would likely have helped to eliminate even more cultural barriers that Mr. Singh faced during his visit. But what ultimately mattered was that someone *listened* to Mr. Singh, not just to his spoken words, but to his unspoken fears and hesitations. I didn't have to be Punjabi Sikh to listen, though our shared Desi culture and Indian roots did help me better understand where his fears were coming from. My experiences and exposure to Sikh culture allowed me to more readily put myself in the shoes of Mr. Singh and mentally question, "How would I feel if I was wearing a turban and was asked to change into a surgical mask in the middle of the waiting room?"

I suppose Mr. Singh must have appreciated our efforts nonetheless, because for the rest of his visit, he was beaming. He insisted that I stay in the patient room during the doctor's visit, even though I knew no Punjabi and our knowledge of Hindi was mutually weak and we had a Punjabi interpreter on the phone. After the doctor left, Mr. Singh asked that I do his blood draw and give him his vaccinations, even though I was not on shift for clinical duties that day. He insisted that I call him "Uncle," even though we only met an hour ago.

Though I was not Punjabi, Mr. Singh saw me as his advocate—as someone who would guide him in this unfamiliar setting, voice his apprehensions, and navigate his cultural beliefs and practices with familiarity and ease. And though I was not Sikh, we both shared the culture of our motherland and considered our Indian roots to be a significant part of our identity. He sought a shore of familiarity in this ocean of unknown, and I was the first he had found.

* * *

Patient comfort has always been an integral part of healthcare, but how much of a role does familiarity play in breeding comfort? In 2020, Cynthia Wensley and Ann McKillop, both faculty members at the University of Auckland School of Nursing, set out to create a framework to define *comfort*. After reviewing over sixty-two different studies and conducting twenty-five semi-structured interviews among a sample of culturally diverse patients (including Maori and Pacific Islander populations), Wensley and McKillop developed a framework to represent patients' perspectives of comfort in an acute care setting. This framework, called Comfort ALways Matters (or CALM for short), analyzes the different factors that play a role in influencing the comfort a patient experiences.

According to the patient data they collected, Wensley and McKillop identified four different types of comfort patients experience:

1. Relief from emotional and physical pain or distress
2. Feeling safe, stronger, and more positive
3. Feeling confident, in control, and autonomous in receiving treatment
4. Feeling cared for, valued, and connecting positively to the people and place

The CALM framework suggests that family, staff, clinical environment, and even the patient themselves play a role in maximizing the level of comfort the patient ultimately experiences. One of the primary reasons patients cited as a reason for experiencing maximum comfort was *cultural connectedness*, or "the feeling that one's cultural norms and values were understood and respected by others." Patients perceive cultural connectedness when they observe culturally diverse staff working together to care for patients, quality of communication between staff and families, and availability of cultural support staff. As one Maori patient in the study shared, "I identified with [the nurse] for being from the same place as me, somebody from home. Being Maori and him coming to talk to me, it made a big difference...it was uplifting."

There was truth to the CALM framework, and I started to notice it in my own personal encounters as well. Whenever I make an effort to greet our clinic's Hindi-speaking patients in their own language, I am met with affectionate smiles and hand gestures that say, "Bless you Dear." My Hindi isn't great, but I'd like to think it's my effort to connect with them that counts.

My colleagues at work have started to follow suit. Recently we have been seeing a lot of elderly Hindu Indian and Nepali patients in our clinic, many of whom have been unable to return to their home country due to COVID-19 travel restrictions. They are understandably stressed and confused about the many aspects of living in a new country and culture, not to mention scared about the prospect of navigating our healthcare system without any insurance. Our front desk staff greets them with a "namaste" and folds their hands together in respect when they check in. Our patients beam with joy, and it sets a positive tone for the rest of their visit. It helps them feel more welcome in an otherwise scary and unfamiliar environment.

The impact clinical staff can have on a patient's perception of comfort, and as a result on their subsequent healing and wellness, is enormous. This impact is enhanced in an environment where patients perceive their cultural norms and values are understood and respected, and this was the perception of our clinic I hoped Mr. Singh would walk away with.

As I walked Mr. Singh out of the clinic at the end of his visit, he stopped in his tracks when we reached the door. He turned back around to face me, he cupped his hand over my head, and he said, "Bless you, my daughter."

In interacting with and taking care of Mr. Singh, I couldn't help but wonder if he would have responded just as warmly had I not been familiar with his culture's practices. I decided to ask my friend and fellow-Telugu American, Prithvi Mavuri, about what he believed to be the role of cultural familiarity in patient care. Prithvi is a third-year Internal Medicine resident at Augusta Hospital in Georgia. Though he grew up here in the US, his roots are based in the Telugu state of Andhra Pradesh in India, where both of our families are from. With such a strong attachment and appreciation for his Telugu culture through language, food, movies, dance, and even a podcast series he hosts about the Telugu diaspora experience, I knew Prithvi would be the best person to ask about this. I wanted to know if he believed his attachment to Indian culture led his Indian patients to be more receptive to him. In response, Prithvi shared with me a particularly memorable patient encounter he had experienced some time ago in his earlier years of residency.

Being the overnight resident responsible for the eighty patients across the different floors meant Prithvi was constantly bombarded with page after page. *Anemia, Room 208; Cellulitis, Room 310; Hypoglycemia, Room 232;* and so on and so forth. Then, Prithvi got another page: "Patient in 215 with massive GI bleed. Please come and evaluate." Prithvi looked at the patient's records.

```
Patient Name: Subbarao Nandagiri
Age: 72
```

This was Prithvi's first ever Telugu patient. As Prithvi gathered the patient's charts and made his way towards Room 215, one of the nurses stopped him at the door.

She leaned in and whispered annoyedly, "This family's a little much. There's a whole gang of them there."

Prithvi nodded and walked in, and sure enough the whole family was there. Subbarao *garu* (a term of respect for elders) was on the patient bed, crowded by his three sons and wife in the small patient room. And yet, Prithvi was not the least perturbed by this. He smiled warmly at them all and folded his hands together.

"*Namaskaram andi, ela unnaru?* How are you doing?"

The moment he greeted them in Telugu, something in the room changed. There was a new feeling of comfort in the air, a feeling of ease and safety. It was the feeling that came with being surrounded by their own people. As Prithvi described it, it was an acknowledgment of the fact that "*mana vaallu ocharu*," that our people, our own Telugu people, have come to take care of us.

Prithvi, unlike the nurse outside, understood why the entire family wished to stay with Subbarao *garu* in the room. He understood what others perhaps saw as over-bearing was really how his sons showed care and filial affection towards their father. It was a part of the Telugu culture. When your mother or father is hurt, of course you're going to be there for them to make sure they're okay. As Telugus ourselves, Prithvi or I would do the same if we were in these sons' situation.

On top of this, Subbarao *garu* was new to the US. He didn't know what the norms and practices of this country were, let alone of this country's healthcare system. As Prithvi had observed from his years in India, healthcare in India is completely different. In India, the doctor is considered God, and whatever they tell you is what you do, no questions asked. It's very much a paternalistic patient-doctor relationship. In the US however, you have the opportunity (and are often even encouraged) to do your own research and question the doctor and push back a little bit. The adherence is a bit more lenient.

In India, you pay for your doctor's visits upfront, not having to worry about co-pays and incompatible insurance plans typical of American healthcare. Meanwhile in the US, there are a lot of protective measures, many of which Eastern medicine would tend to consider excess. People don't go to rehab post-hospitalization in India. They go home after being in the hospital for so long, and they reunite with their family and loved ones.

As an Indian patient receiving care in the American healthcare system, there is no way Subbarao *garu* would have known all of this, unless someone told him and assured him it would all be okay. That was perhaps why he and his sons felt so understood when Prithvi spoke to them. Prithvi not only knew the language, but he also recognized the cultural barriers the family experienced in addition to Subbarao *garu's* existing medical complications. Even though this was a strange situation in a strange environment for Subbarao *garu* and his family, it was mutually understood that Prithvi would walk them through this unfamiliarity. He would be there to help them feel safe and understood.

It was the same thing when Prithvi would meet with a Black patient, and his Black colleague was also with him in the room. There are three Black physicians in Prithvi's residency program, and this is something they share with

Prithvi time and time again. The change in body language, the jargon they speak, the code-switch that happens—everything changes when the patients see that their doctor is also Black. There's an instant shift in the ambience. And when Black doctors see their Black patients, they understand what life is like at home for the patient. They know how they speak. They know how they eat. They know the cultural norm that looks down upon Black men seeking mental health support. The doctor connects with the patient upon a shared culture, and the patient feels a lot more comfortable sharing his information with the doctor, confident that this time someone will understand him and what he is going through.

In fact, several researchers at the University of Miami recently discovered that having a Black doctor reduces the pain and anxiety experienced by Black patients compared to having a non-Black doctor. By measuring the patients' skin conductance response and pulse, the researchers were able to determine the intensity of anxiety and pain experienced by the patients. As lead author of the study Steven Anderson shares, "Physician diversity initiatives are often seen as beneficial for improving patient comfort and satisfaction, but with our study, we have evidence that there may be direct health consequences to not having a diverse workforce as well."

Regardless of what race, ethnicity, or culture the patient belongs to, we see the same pattern again and again: familiarity breeds comfort. Having someone who understands the patient's culture and offers a feeling of familiarity is automatically able to create a more welcoming and comforting environment for the patient.

Whether it was Prithvi speaking in Telugu to assure his patient, me helping Mr. Singh find a way to accommodate his turban and mask, or the nurse speaking to his Maori patient in his own language, we as providers and cultural brokers are uniquely positioned to offer our patients the comfort of familiarity in an otherwise scary and foreign environment.

CHAPTER 3

THE CHAMELEON EFFECT

"Treatment is not just limited to the medical therapy you provide. It includes how you speak to them and how you connect with them."

— PRITHVI MAVURI, INTERNAL MEDICINE
RESIDENT AT AUGUSTA UNIVERSITY HOSPITAL

The holiday season had arrived, and it was a particularly busy Monday afternoon at the clinic. Every single patient room was full, and us MAs (medical assistants) were running up and down the hallway, our hands full with labs to run, urine to collect, blood to draw, vaccines to inject, and patients to discharge.

Room One had been occupied for over an hour and a half now. The green light was off, meaning the doctor was done seeing the patient. The head MA had already run the labs and drawn blood for Room One. This patient was definitely ready to be discharged.

I knocked on the door and poked my head in. It was Michael, a middle-aged Indian man who had been coming to our clinic for a little over four months now for abdominal pain and hypertension. Apart from a couple of hellos and goodbyes, we never had the opportunity to share a conversation. I stepped into the room and asked him, "Hi Michael, is there anything that I can help you out with?"

He nodded and began to speak in his steady accented English, "I don't know how to say this or who to tell this to, but I know why my BP has been so high lately."

He began to tell me about his fear of being diagnosed with colon cancer. "I can't tell anyone at home about it. I'm the head of my family. My daughter is getting married soon, and I can't let them worry about me right now. I have to stay strong for them."

Michael was an undocumented immigrant who fled from India almost ten years ago to seek asylum in the US. As he worked and earned money here in the city, he financially supported his family who lived on the other side of the world in Bangalore. Though he spoke to his family over the phone every single day and missed them dearly, he couldn't bear to share this piece of news with them. He had kept his pending diagnosis and the associated emotions bottled up inside, never having an opportunity to open up with anyone about them. His stress about his diagnosis had been impacting his health and, as we soon learned, manifesting itself in the form of severe hypertensive episodes.

"Did you tell the doctor that you've been feeling this way?" I asked.

He shook his head. "I feel you will understand so I am telling you first."

He didn't choose to tell the energetic and personable attending physician who saw him for his appointment. He didn't choose to tell the sweet and motherly head MA who drew his blood. He didn't choose to tell any of the other staff or physicians that were there. But he chose to tell me, a young and inexperienced new hire who had barely even spoken to him before. The reason? I was the only one among our staff who was Indian.

What was strange was that we didn't even speak the same Indian language. I spoke Telugu while he spoke Kannada. I was Hindu while he was Catholic. I was born and raised in California while he was born and raised in Karnataka. We didn't even share the same skin color. Though we were both considered "brown," I was dark skinned while he was light skinned. And yet, we understood each other. We both shared the culture of our mother country. And in our culture, men didn't always have the liberty to share their emotions and internal struggles with others. I saw my dad in him.

I couldn't help but wonder. Did my Indian-ness really made that much of a difference for this patient?

As it turned out, I wasn't alone in my inquiry. Dr. Majid Jalil and Professor Rosslynne Freeman explored this very issue in their 2001 research study about the role of the provider's culture in the patient-provider relationship. How exactly does one's culture affect this relationship? And does the successful outcome of the consultation depend on the shared culture of the doctor and patient?

Jalil and Freeman observed, recorded, and analyzed over 150 patient consultations in both Pakistan and London, where doctors worked in "cross-culture" and "same-culture" contexts. After conducting interviews of both doctors and patients in these contexts and analyzing the resulting themes from these consultations, Jalil and Freeman made an important discovery. As it turns out, culture *does* indeed affect the outcome of the consultation, and as a result plays a significant role in the quality of care the patient receives.

For example, one consistent theme Jalil and Freeman found was Pakistani patients held starkly different expectations for their doctors compared to their British counterparts. They believed this difference in expectations emerged from the difference in cultural dimensions between the two cultures.

In 1980, the Dutch management researcher Geert Hofstede developed a revolutionary theory, which he coined as his Cultural Dimensions Theory, to better understand cultural differences across countries and determine the impact of these cultural dimensions on cross-cultural communication. One such cultural dimension of Hofstede's Cultural Dimensions Theory, called *power distance*, measures the degree to which hierarchy and inequality is accepted among members of society.

Jalil and Freeman found the Pakistani patients, who came from a higher power distance culture according to Hofstede's theory, accepted the doctor-patient hierarchy more readily and preferred their doctor to be more authoritative and paternalistic. On the other hand, the British patients, who came from a lower power distance culture, preferred that their doctor was more open and collaborative with them.

The most interesting part of the study, however, was how the doctors were able to accommodate these distinct and conflicting cultural expectations of their patients. Jalil and Freeman were impressed to find their Pakistani colleagues who worked in London had learned to adapt and code-switch between the differing cultural expectations of their Pakistani and British patients alike. Like chameleons, they effortlessly moved between consultation styles to fit the expectations and needs of both their Pakistani and British patients. Through their study, Jalil and Freeman were able to demonstrate that a provider can serve as a reliable cultural broker for their patients when they both have an existing familiarity with their patient's cultural needs *and* put in the effort to understand and accommodate those needs.

* * *

How exactly does a provider *"chameleon"* themselves to fit the cultural needs of their patient? And how does cultural familiarity make this process easier? Dr. Chaitanya Patel (name changed upon request), a first-year Internal Medicine resident, has found himself in this "chameleon" role quite often as an Indian American doctor.

Chaitanya works at the Augusta University Hospital, which stands in the heart of the city of Augusta, Georgia. Augusta is a decently sized city with a fairly diverse population, which means Chaitanya often sees patients from a variety of different cultural backgrounds. According to Chaitanya, there's the roots of Augusta, the old white wealthy families that have lived in the area for generations. Then there's the military base, which brings in a lot of military and veteran folk. There's also a couple of cybersecurity centers as well as a large nuclear plant, which brings in more of the younger and foreign-born engineers. This is where the hospital ends up getting a lot of its Indian and Asian patient population from.

It was a warm and sunny morning, and the Augusta University ICU was bustling with patients as usual.

Chaitanya had just signed on for his morning shift. The overnight resident handed off the previous night's patients to Chaitanya, presenting the cases one by one. *GI bleed in 208. Cellulitis in 212. Hypoglycemia in 213. Lung contusion in 215. Anemia in 218.*

He paused and looked up at Chaitanya at the mention of "anemia."

"The anemia patient. She's a hard one. She's not giving me any info to work with."

The overnight team found that she had extremely low hemoglobin levels upon admission into the ICU, which meant that her blood wasn't transporting enough oxygen to the rest of her body. If left untreated, her severe anemia could result in multi-organ failure, cognitive impairment, and even death. In order to properly treat her anemia, the medical team first had to identify the cause behind it.

They began by screening for heavy blood loss, be it through trauma, internal bleeding, or bloody vomit and bowel movements. Next, they looked for nutritional deficiencies, namely iron-deficiencies, that might be preventing her blood from properly carrying the oxygen it was supposed to. Finally, they looked at any medications, liver or spleen issues, or other systemic conditions that would cause hemolysis, or the breaking open of red blood cells in the body.

The good news was there was a set list of questions to ask and tests to order. The bad news was the cause could be literally anything, from iron-deficiency to kidney failure to blood thinner use. If they didn't get the answers they were looking for, the patient could very well die. The team had no idea as to why this patient had such low hemoglobin, but they couldn't go forward with the diagnosis until the patient shared her side of the story. They were in a race against time.

Chaitanya nodded as the night resident handed over the patient files. *Priya Agrawal*, the name on the file read.

"Does she speak Hindi?" Chaitanya asked.

"Not sure, I guess so?"

"Perhaps I can help interpret for the patient, maybe then she'll be more comfortable sharing the info in her own language," Chaitanya offered.

The resident shrugged dismissively. "Good luck with that."

A few hours later, Chaitanya and Anna, another of his fellow residents, walked into Room 218 together. Anna would serve as the primary physician for this patient, while Chaitanya would take on the role of Hindi interpreter for the visit.

The patient lay on the bed with an IV in her left arm connected to several bags of fluids. She looked relatively young, probably in her thirties or so. Her black hair was mussed up against the thin papery pillowcase, and beads of sweat dripped down the sides of her tired face.

"Nice to meet you Priya," Anna waved. My name is Dr. Wang and this is Dr. Patel."

Priya smiled weakly at Anna. She looked over at Chaitanya and nodded.

"Hi Priya, *aap kaise hai?* How are you?" Chaitanya asked.

"*Main theek hoon.* I'm okay."

"It's good to hear that you're doing better than last night. What happened yesterday that brought you to the ICU?"

Priya looked at Chaitanya to interpret for her into Hindi. He nodded. She began to narrate yesterday's events, starting with the extreme bout of dizziness and headache that had hit her yesterday afternoon. Her heart was beating especially fast, and she felt like the air was being sucked out of her lungs. Though her face felt hot and sweaty, her hands and feet were cold. Her symptoms kept getting worse. After an hour or so, she passed out in the middle of her living room.

"Based on your blood tests we ran yesterday, it looks like your hemoglobin levels are extremely low, which means your body isn't getting enough oxygen. In order to give you the right treatment, we need to figure out why your hemoglobin is so low," Anna explained. Chaitanya repeated it in Hindi, and Priya nodded in acknowledgement.

"Have you ever experienced something like this before?"

Priya paused for a moment before replying, "*Itna bura kabhi nahi.* Never this bad."

"Do you have any history of heart or kidney problems? Or anyone in your family?"

Priya shook her head.

Anna continued her assessment of each of the body systems, running through her checklist of questions to ask. Any recent trauma? Any heavy bleeding? Priya answered each question with the assistance of Chaitanya's Hindi interpretation. When Anna reached the gynecological system, she asked Priya, "How have your periods been recently?"

Priya suddenly grew quiet, her eyes wide. She looked down at her hands, averting her gaze from Anna and Chaitanya.

"It's okay, you can tell us," Anna said softly. "Have your recent periods been irregular?"

Priya looked to Chaitanya with an uncomfortable look in her eyes. And that's when Chaitanya understood.

In India, the woman is told to sit alone during her period, away from the rest of the family, until her bleeding stops. She is not allowed to enter the kitchen or touch any cooking utensils. She is not allowed to touch the laundry. She is not allowed to eat certain foods. She is not allowed to go out. If she asks why, she is simply told she must respect "age-old tradition" and breaking this tradition would bring "taboo."

However, this taboo surrounding menstruation and women's health is a relatively recent development in the vast historical timeline of the Indian subcontinent. Sinu Joseph, a menstrual hygiene educator and women's health advocate from Kerala, explores the ancient origins of menstrual practices and their eventual corruption in her recent book *Rtu Vidya: Ancient Science Behind Menstrual Practices.* In ancient India, a woman on her period was considered to be the Divine Mother, a living goddess who carried the seed of the unborn. As such, the woman's family would take over her household responsibilities in order to let her rest. Her period was one of the few times she was presented with the opportunity to relax her mind and restore her health and strength by taking time and space to herself.

But sadly, over time, society has taken this ritual and turned it into a shameful act. A woman's relief from chores was turned into banishment from the household. Her divine status during her period was turned into a lowly rank of impurity and inferiority. What began as a way to give women a break from their daily responsibilities eventually turned into a taboo that saw women and their periods as filthy and impure. As Sinu quotes in her book's epigraph, "What is pure we do not touch. And what we do not touch, we call it a taboo."

Now because of the corruption of these original ancient practices, periods have turned into a taboo in today's society. Discussion about anything relating to women's hygiene or reproductive health is looked down upon. To openly discuss one's menstruation with the opposite gender? Unthinkable.

Chaitanya understood Priya's dilemma. His mother, his sister, and his wife would have reacted in the same way if they were in Priya's position. But this situation was different. Chaitanya and Anna were Priya's doctors, and they needed to know these details in order to provide her with the proper treatment and care.

"I can understand how you must feel, Priya. *Main samajhata hoon.* But this is an issue of your health. In situations like these, we sometimes have to set aside our cultural taboos and traditions for the sake of our health and betterment."

Priya lifted her gaze from her hands and looked at Chaitanya. The resident last night asked her the same questions as Anna and Chaitanya, but she was not in a place to share any information with him. He was not Indian. He was not a woman. He did not know Hindi. He did not understand the cultural stigma she struggled with in order to discuss her period so openly. How then could she share such sensitive information about herself with someone who didn't understand her?

But Chaitanya and Anna on the other hand, she could share with. Anna was a woman. She had the lived experience of periods. And Chaitanya, though he was male, understood the cultural taboos she faced. Not to mention, he knew Hindi. She knew enough English to get by, but she didn't know enough to be able to explain everything clearly to the doctors. Hindi was by far her preferred language and having someone in the room who spoke her language and understood her culture was important to her.

After some hesitation, Priya nodded. "*Bataungi*. I will tell you."

Priya shared she had been experiencing particularly heavy bleeding over the last few months, and she had been especially feeling dizzy and sweaty over the last few weeks. She wasn't on any form of birth control, nor did she have any previous indications that would point to her heavy menstrual bleeding.

Anna and Chaitanya looked at each other and nodded.

"Thank you so much for sharing this," Anna said. "We can understand how difficult this must be for you, but this was exactly the information we needed to figure out what was causing your anemia."

Chaitanya added, "And Priya, rest assured that your information will be kept completely confidential and private. Whatever you told us here is just for us to discuss, not for anyone else. *Kisi ko pata nahi chalega.*"

With this information, Anna and Chaitanya were able to get OB-GYN specialists involved and manage her care more accurately. If Chaitanya wasn't there to offer Hindi interpretation and help facilitate the much-needed patient-doctor conversation, it likely would have taken a lot longer to find the cause of Priya's issue, which could have dangerously affected her health.

* * *

We see this trend repeatedly: familiarity breeds better outcomes. Familiarity and comfort are what enables the provider to work toward understanding the barriers their patient faces. They increase the patient's willingness to disclose information, seek help, and participate in treatment rather than pulling away. "At the end of the day, it's all about the confidence a patient has in their doctor," explains Dr. Sirisha Narayana, a Telugu-American Internal Medicine hospitalist at UCSF. "It's about how I care for them and their acute medical issue, so whatever I can do to ally with my patients plays a key part in building this confidence." When the doctor is able to offer this comfort of familiarity, the patient's confidence and trust in their doctor is enhanced.

I first learned of Sirisha through a podcast episode on *The Nocturnists*, in which she discusses the intersection of her many identities including that of being a physician, being Telugu-American, and being a woman. In the episode, she shares a gripping story about a phenomenon she calls the "Aunty effect."

One day, an elderly Indian woman (let's call her Ms. Jain) was admitted into the hospital with a urinary tract infection. She was confused and wasn't particularly responsive. Sirisha and the rest of the team were rubbing her sternum, which is a pain-inducing technique used to assess one's consciousness by rubbing one's knuckles in a grinding motion on the chest bone. As they performed the sternal rub, they screamed into her ear, "Ms. Jain, can you hear us?"

Sirisha's intern, a young woman also of Indian descent, paused for a minute before approaching the patient. Then she calmly bent over, shook the patient's arm, and said very assertively, "Aunty!"

In many South Asian cultures, older men and women are referred to as Uncle and Aunty out of respect (even though they're not actually related by blood). It's one of the most second nature parts of being Indian to say, "Yes Aunty" or "Thanks Uncle," but it was still surprising to Sirisha to hear her intern call this woman "Aunty." As a doctor in a hospital setting, it felt strange to Sirisha to place the identity of "Aunty" upon her patient. And yet, she wouldn't have thought twice in any other context.

Sirisha looked at her intern with a raised eyebrow, to which the intern responded, "What? It's probably comforting to her!" The intern tried again, shaking the patients arm and loudly calling, "Aunty!"

And that's when Ms. Jain turned to the intern and said, "Whaaat!"

Sirisha was shook. This patient, for whom screaming into her ear and performing a sternal rub was insufficient, responded to the intern calling her "Aunty."

This intersectionality of identities, this crossing of her physician self and Indian self, was a situation Sirisha rarely found herself in. Perhaps that was why Sirisha's initial reaction told her that calling her patient "Aunty" wasn't appropriate. And yet, the feelings of positivity, safety, and confidence the intern was able to offer her patient with this simple word "Aunty" were insurmountable. By adapting her ways to fit her patient's cultural expectations, even if at odds with typical hospital culture, the intern was able to revive her patient.

A few months later, Sirisha was taking care of another elderly Indian woman who also came into the hospital in a confused and unresponsive state. This time, Sirisha decided to use the same trick that her intern had used with Ms. Jain.

"Aunty!" Sirisha called to her.

To her surprise, it worked yet again. In fact, the patient responded far better to "Aunty" than to the sternal rub. The "Aunty" effect was beyond medical science, but it worked. "Aunty" was the expression of cultural familiarity, the same factor that Dr. Jalil and Prof. Freeman found in their research to be vital to the patient's quality of care, and the same factor that allowed Chaitanya and Anna to provide the necessary treatment to their Hindi-speaking patient.

The best part? Sirisha's entire team, all four tall white men, started calling the patient "Aunty." The intern was right. Calling the patient "Aunty" probably helped her realize she was safe, and she was among her people.

CHAPTER 4

KEEPING SECRETS AND BREAKING TRUST

"A breach in trust brings mistrust, followed by a multitude of troubles."

— PAVAN MISHRA, *COINMAN: AN UNTOLD CONSPIRACY*

In 1932, in Macon County, Alabama, the US Public Health Service (USPHS) began a six-month clinical study to observe the natural progression of untreated syphilis, a chronic bacterial infection that is either sexually transmitted or passed congenitally from mother to baby (CDC, 2021). We now know that syphilis progresses in stages, with symptoms ranging from mild sores and body rashes all the way to permanent damage to the nervous system and heart (Mayo Clinic, 2021).

In collaboration with the Tuskegee Institute of Alabama, the USPHS investigators who were in charge of this study enrolled 600 impoverished African American sharecroppers in Macon County, all male, to participate in the study as clinical subjects. Of the men, 399 had latent syphilis, while 201 had no infection and were used as a control group (Brown, 2017). As incentive to participate in the study, the USPHS promised these men they would receive free medical care from the US federal government (CDC, 2021).

Unfortunately, they didn't keep their promise. Instead of informing the subjects of their syphilis diagnosis, the clinicians and investigators simply told the subjects that they were being treated for "bad blood," a colloquial term for a set of conditions that included fatigue, anemia, and others. At this time, "bad blood" was a leading cause of death among the African American community in the South. Charles Pollard, one of the few survivors, recalled: "All I knew was that they just kept saying I had the bad blood—they never mentioned syphilis to me. Not even once" (Brown, 2017).

In addition, the clinicians disguised placebos and diagnostic methods as "treatments" for their disease. According to Susan Reverby's 2009 book, *Examining Tuskegee*, they used incredibly toxic compounds such as bismuth, mercurial ointments, and Salvarsan "606" (an arsenic compound) as treatments. While these compounds were somewhat effective in killing the bacteria that caused syphilis, they invariably poisoned the patient in the process due to their toxic nature, producing undesirable side effects including liver and brain damage (Williams, 2009).

In order to continue receiving diagnostic data for their study, clinicians misled subjects into receiving repeated spinal taps (Brandt, 1978). The spinal tap is a procedure in which a needle is inserted between two lumbar vertebrae of the spine in order to retrieve a sample of cerebrospinal fluid. These procedures were not only painful and dangerous to these patients, but more importantly they were non-therapeutic, meaning there was no benefit to the patient's recovery in receiving a spinal tap.

Though the subjects were told the study would only last six months, it actually continued for another forty years under the guidance of several USPHS supervisors. The investigators could have chosen to treat all the patients at the end of the six-month period and close off the study. But because their ulterior motive was to observe the natural course of syphilis, the USPHS continued the study without ever informing the test subjects about what was going on (CDC, 2021).

By 1947, fifteen years after the start of the study, penicillin had become widely available and was deemed the primary treatment for syphilis (Gelpi, 2015). With the support of federal government funding, rapid treatment centers were established all over the country in order to eradicate the disease, even in Macon County. However, the subjects of the study were never offered penicillin treatment, nor were they ever informed that penicillin was even a treatment that was widely available. Penicillin, as well as any information about it, was withheld from the subjects. In case they did find out about the treatment, the subjects were prevented from accessing these penicillin treatment programs that were being offered to their neighbors and fellow Macon County residents.

A February 1992 story about the study was featured on ABC's *Prime Time Live*, in which Dr. Sidney Olansky, the USPHS director from 1950-1957, was asked about the penicillin treatment information that was withheld from the study's participants. On air, he replied: "The fact that they were illiterate was helpful, too, because they couldn't read the newspapers. If they were not, as things moved on, they might have been reading newspapers and seen what was going on" (Thomas, 2000).

A few of the study's subjects went on to join the army during WWII, where they were able to receive penicillin treatment and were cured of syphilis as a result. When they returned to Macon County after the war, they told their friends and fellow study participants about how they were treated with penicillin and were cured of the "bad blood." They tried to help the other study participants get access to penicillin treatment, but to no avail. None of the hospitals in the area would treat these test subjects because they were blacklisted. Their names were on a list that stated they should not receive treatment because they were participants of the study (Reverby, 2009).

A number of individuals, including a venereal-disease investigator for the USPHS named Peter Buxtun, expressed to their superiors their criticism and disdain for the many breaches of ethical scientific practice this study employed. "I didn't want to believe it," Buxtun shared. "This was the Public Health Service. We didn't do things like that." (Heller, 1997). But despite the concerns raised by Buxtun and others, the study received the unequivocal support of the US Centers for Disease Control and Prevention (CDC) which insisted the study was to be continued until completion, or in other words, until every single subject had died and been autopsied.

On November 16, 1972, the study was brought to an abrupt end when Peter Buxtun leaked its horrific details to the press. The CDC and USPHS were under extreme public pressure to discontinue the study following the press leak. Upon determining that the test subjects were never informed of the study's actual purpose, a congressionally appointed Health Advisory Panel determined the study to be immoral and medically invalid, and ordered the termination of the study (CDC, 2021). The revelation of this study led to the creation of the Belmont Report, which now serves as the guiding rulebook for the execution of clinical studies and protection of its participants from immoral conduct.

By the end of the study in 1972, a full four decades later, only seventy-four of the original 600 test subjects were alive. Of the original 399 men with syphilis, twenty-eight died of the disease, one hundred died of related complications, forty had wives who were infected, and nineteen bore children who were born with congenital syphilis (CDC, 2021).

This study, often referred to as the "Tuskegee Syphilis Experiment," became a seminal moment in history highlighting the extent of exploitation of African American communities by government officials, public health organizations, medical professionals, and many others. Given the extent of this historic exploitation, it's no wonder the trust of the African American community toward healthcare has broken, and so many from impoverished Black communities are reluctant to seek routine preventative healthcare. A 1999 survey showed that 80 percent of African American men believed the subjects in the Tuskegee study had been intentionally injected with syphilis by the USPHS (Katz, 2008). Additionally, this distrust of the government, due in part to the Tuskegee study, contributed to people's belief that the US government had deliberately introduced the HIV virus into Black communities as part of yet another "scientific study."

To this day, we see the effects of these historical exploitations on our African American patients. Earlier this year, our clinic's social worker was telling me about one of our patients she spoke to recently about insurance options. This woman, who had just turned sixty-five years old, had lived through a significant part of the Tuskegee study and had seen the aftermath of its effects on her family and her community. As a result, she came to develop a strong mistrust of the system, and she didn't want to apply for Medi-Cal or any other government benefits. Even when the social worker explained to the woman that there was nothing to fear and that Healthy San Francisco (a San-Francisco based insurance plan) was a safe non-federal option that she could opt for, the woman refused vehemently. She would rather go without insurance and forego her routine primary care than to give her personal details to the institutions that had exploited her people.

According to a December 2020 Kaiser Family Foundation poll, over one-third of African American adults in the US were unwilling to receive a COVID vaccine due to mistrust in the medical system and fears about vaccine safety (Hamel, 2020). Titilayo (Titi) Mabogunje, a good friend of mine from college, is currently a research assistant at Tufts University where she works to understand the reasons behind this mistrust. Born in England and raised in Nigeria, Titi has seen first-hand what makes a "healthy and wealthy nation" and what is needed to improve healthcare delivery among marginalized populations. "Science is so messed up," Titi lamented as we discussed the implications of racial mistrust in the present-day health system. "The Tuskegee Syphilis

Experiment is a reminder that this country will not hesitate to use minority populations as guinea pigs." Titi hopes to use her lived experiences as a cultural broker to return to Nigeria and practice as a physician.

It's not easy to undo decades, even centuries, of exploitation and damage. This mistrust in the system is so deeply engrained that it requires the work of trusted individuals from the community to serve as agents of change and advocate for these historically marginalized communities. These agents of change, these cultural brokers, have not only built deep connections and garnered trust within their communities, but have also worked to understand the cultural expectations of both marginalized and mainstream communities in order to effortlessly navigate between the two. Cultural brokers like Titi that understand the mistrust and reservations of their communities are uniquely positioned to serve as a facilitator for rebuilding trust in the system. In order to rebuild trust, cultural brokers must be made a bigger priority.

Historical mistrust is only one example of the many ways in which the trust between patient and provider can be compromised. We just as frequently see instances in which patients lose trust in doctors as a whole due to the loss of confidentiality. A successful patient-provider relationship is built upon mutual respect and trust. The provider is expected to uphold certain standards of ethics and integrity, and in return the patient is expected to be honest about their personal medical history. But when the provider's respect for their patient is lost, so is the patient's trust in their doctor...and eventually in all doctors.

Donya Tserendolgor, our clinic's volunteer Mongolian interpreter, has worked in healthcare for over two decades. Over the course of her time in the US, she has seen her fair share of cases in which the patient did not trust the doctor due to previous negative experiences surrounding healthcare. When she can, Donya works to fill that role of being a cultural broker for these patients to help them rebuild trust in the doctors and medical system that are there to take care of them. Donya shared a few stories with me from her time working as a Mongolian interpreter at the city hospital.

A sixty-seven-year-old Mongolian woman (let's call her Enkhee Batsuh) came in one Wednesday morning for a general checkup and Pap smear. The Pap smear is a method used to screen for cervical cancer by scraping a few cells from the cervix for examination under a microscope. It is commonly recommended in the US that individuals begin screening every few years starting at the age of twenty-one. In Mongolia however, Pap smears were performed at much lower rates. In fact, only 30 percent of all women between the ages of fifteen to forty-nine had ever been screened (HPV Information Center, 2019). Mrs. Batsuh was a part of the majority. She had never received a Pap smear before, and this was her first one.

After collecting her vitals, the nurse gave Mrs. Batsuh a patient gown to change into and instructed her to wait in the exam room. Mrs. Batsuh stripped down, wore the gown, and sat on the patient table. Mrs. Batsuh looked around the room. On the pink paper-towel-covered counter lay an assortment of various medical instruments and tools: a small examination flashlight, a plastic speculum, a plastic spatula, a thin brush, a small cylindrical container, some packets of lubricating gel, and a short strip of orange pH paper.

Some moments later, the doctor walked in. Mrs. Batsuh was not comfortable with communicating in English, so Donya also entered the room to serve as a Mongolian interpreter between Mrs. Batsuh and the doctor.

"Nice to meet you Mrs. Batsuh," the doctor greeted her with a warm smile.

"*Enkhee,*" the patient replied.

Donya leaned in and whispered to the doctor to call her Enkhee instead of Mrs. Batsuh. Unlike in Western culture where we refer to people using their last names as a form of respect (e.g., Mr. Smith or Mrs. Doe), last names are never used in Mongolian culture. The father's first name is taken as the individual's last name, and therefore must not be spoken aloud out of respect for the father. As such, many Mongolians only use their first name, with the exception of government documentation and other circumstances that require their last name to be used.

"My apologies Enkhee. Please lie down," the doctor instructed as she slipped on a pair of nitrile gloves.

"*Khevteerei,*" Donya translated.

Enkhee put her head on the pillow and scooted down so that her hips were lined up with the edge of the table. The doctor pulled out the stirrups from the sides of the table and Donya guided Enkhee's feet into the stirrups.

The doctor sat on a low rolling stool that placed her at eye level with Enkhee's cervix. She lifted up Enkhee's gown, turned on the speculum light, and gently coerced the speculum into the vaginal canal. Enkhee shut her eyes tight and balled her fists. The doctor peered closely as she tried rocking the speculum up and down. No luck. Enkhee let out a small grunt.

"I'm sorry," the doctor said as she removed the speculum and tried reinserting at a slightly higher angle.

"Ow!" Enkhee yelled.

After several unsuccessful attempts to readjust the speculum, the doctor placed a drape over Enkhee's legs and told her, "I'll be right back."

"*Ter shuud ergej irne,*" Donya translated.

Enkhee nodded, her eyes still shut tight and her fists balled.

A few minutes later, the doctor walked back into the room accompanied by another doctor. They each took turns sitting on the stool and peering into Enkhee's vaginal opening, readjusting the speculum this way and that. Enkhee let out a shrill cry of pain. The doctors were both perplexed. *Where was her cervix?* They looked over at Donya for any info she might have.

Donya shrugged, "I don't know."

The doctors murmured to each other, and then placed the drape back over Enkhee's legs.

"We apologize for the pain, Enkhee. We will be right back."

"*Bid yag odoo ergej irne,*" Donya translated.

Once the doctors stepped out of the room, Enkhee opened her eyes and motioned for Donya to come close.

"I have to tell you something. *Nadad chamd khelekh züil baina.* Please keep it a secret."

Donya nodded and leaned in.

"I got a cosmetic surgery in Mongolia, right before I moved to the US," Enkhee whispered.

As Donya mentioned to me, cosmetic surgeries of the cervix were extremely popular among women in Mongolia in the 1990s. Women (especially married women who had gone through natural childbirth) would opt for elective surgery to tighten their cervix and vaginal walls so that they could experience a more enjoyable sex life.

Enkhee had told no one about this procedure she received, not her doctor, not her friends, not her family, not even her husband. Back when she was living in Mongolia, a friend of hers had given her a piece of advice:

"Never tell the doctor about your past medical history."

Enkhee had heard horror stories of patients who had shared confidential medical information with their doctors in Mongolia, only to have that information leaked and shared with others in the community and make its way back to the patients. Mongolia is the world's most sparsely populated country (in terms of capita per square mile), due to its dangerous geography and harsh climates. As a result, the communities of people in these areas were small. Donya suspects this was why everyone knew everything about everyone, and why secrets were exceedingly difficult to keep from spreading.

Donya understood exactly what Enkhee was talking about. As a native Mongolian herself, Donya grew up surrounded by this culture of gossip that was rampant within her community. Donya recalls a particular evening from her teenage years when she was sitting with her mom on the verandah, chatting about various things. A few minutes into the conversation, the topic shifted to Donya's friends, specifically her friend Babu.

Donya's mother leaned in with a gleam in her eyes and her hand over her mouth. In a muffled whisper, she said to Donya, "Do you know what happened to Babu's father?"

Donya shook her head no.

"He lost his penis. He had surgery to get it removed."

Donya's cheeks flushed. This was certainly not a topic of conversation she was expecting or hoping to have with her mother, particularly not such a topic about her friend's father.

Donya's mother went on to explain that Babu's father was suffering from penile cancer. The doctors had said that the only way to save his life and prevent the cancer from spreading was to perform a total penectomy, in which the entire penis is removed and a new urinary opening is surgically created in the perineum.

Donya was even more horrified to find out she was one of the last people to have heard this news. The news of Babu's father's surgery had spread like wildfire, and soon enough, every single person in the town knew he no longer had a penis.

Donya imagined what it would be like to be in his position. What if she had breast cancer and received a mastectomy? She would have been mortified to find out the entire town, all her friends, family, peers, acquaintances, and neighbors knew she was wearing a fake breast.

No wonder such fear existed in the Mongolian community. Fear of being open, fear of sharing too much, fear of their private information landing in the wrong ears. They couldn't even trust the doctors to keep their information private, since there were more than enough accounts of doctors chatting it up with family and friends about their patients. "Did you hear Tugi tested positive for syphilis? Did you know Bulga got an abortion? Did I mention Askaa had to get a sperm donation to have babies?"

This was why Mongolians were so incredibly careful about keeping their information private, to the extent they didn't dare share their information with their doctors, the ones responsible for their health. Unlike in the US, doctors in Mongolia were not bound by HIPAA laws. People were hesitant to even go to the doctors to get screened for STDs because of the associated negative stigma, let alone the fear of their diagnosis being shared with others in the community. As a result, there was a raging epidemic of syphilis, gonorrhea, and chlamydia in Mongolia during the 1990s, when the prevalent rates of these diseases almost tripled within the decade (Ebright, 2003).

But for the first time, Enkhee was revealing her secret to Donya, albeit with great fear that her reputation would be ruined if her doctors found out and spread her information to her family and friends.

"I'm scared to tell anyone," Enkhee shared.

"No, no, no!" Donya replied. "You have got the completely wrong message from your friend."

Donya went on to explain to Enkhee about how HIPAA and privacy laws in the US would protect her from having any of her health information revealed to those who did not have her consent. Anyone who violated these privacy laws would be penalized depending on the intent and nature of the violation, with the maximum penalty being upward of $1.5 million per year (Garcia, 2019).

"You have to be open and honest with your doctor," Donya emphasized to Enkhee. "That's the only way they can give you the best care."

Donya, having lived through the same struggles as Enkhee in Mongolia, understood the reason behind

Enkhee's hesitation. But at the same time, Donya's many years of experience of working in healthcare in the US had enabled her to both overcome her own fears and to understand how the culture here differed from the culture back home. Donya's role as a cultural broker was vital to Enkhee's continued trust and health. If anyone, Donya was *the* person to help Enkhee overcome her fears and communicate openly with the doctors.

"So...it is okay to tell the doctor about my cosmetic surgery?" Enkhee asked.

Donya nodded. "They are here to help you, and they can only help you if you are open and honest with them."

A few moments later, the two doctors walked back into the room, scratching their heads. Donya looked at Enkhee, who nodded.

Enkhee then explained to the doctors, with Donya's translation, that she had received a cosmetic surgery back when she was in Mongolia and she was hesitant to share this information due to cultural reasons.

"So that's why there was a scar! We couldn't find the cervix no matter how much we tried," the doctor said. "I'm so sorry, you must have been in so much pain when we were doing the examination."

Donya translated to which Enkhee smiled and nodded in response.

"*Tiim.* Yes."

"In that case, I think we can skip the Pap smear for now."

CHAPTER 5

THE SAFFRON GODDESS

"There's a popular saying among doctors: There's no such thing as alternative medicine; if it works, it's just called medicine."

— ED YONG, *I CONTAIN MULTITUDES: THE MICROBES WITHIN US AND A GRANDER VIEW OF LIFE*

Do no harm. These are the immortal words of the Hippocratic Oath. Kept alive from the White Coat Ceremony at the beginning of a medical student's foray into medicine all the way until the end of the physician's career, this concept of non-maleficence is a defining pillar of medical ethics in Western medicine. In fact, medical ethics in the West is upheld by four such pillars:

1. Autonomy: the individual's right to make decisions for themselves
2. Justice: equal treatment of every individual
3. Beneficence: aiming to always work in the best interest of the patient
4. Non-maleficence: do no harm

Guided by these pillars of medical ethics, the physician must counsel the patient to make an appropriate decision about their health such that it puts them at the least amount of risk and greatest amount of benefit. However, an important yet oft-forgotten part of "do no harm" is recognizing and understanding that different patients might hold different beliefs from providers about what harm means to them. In other words, what a patient sees as beneficial and healthy might actually be seen as harmful by the physician, and vice versa. As Prerna Balasundaram, a graduate of International Affairs at the George Washington Elliott School, explains on the *Matters of State* podcast, "Cultural competency is an essential component of a doctor being able to do no harm. If a doctor wants to adhere to their code of medical ethics, they must be well versed in cultural competency."

Prerna shares the story of a Western OB-GYN doctor she interviewed who practiced for some months in Haiti where birthing practices are incredibly different from the US. After giving birth, Haitian women sit on steaming pots filled with local herbs as per custom. This doctor was horrified to find that so many women who sat on these pots were getting second-degree burns on their pelvic area from the steam and required immediate medical attention as a result. This birthing practice violates the fourth pillar of non-maleficence in Western medical ethics, and therefore could reasonably be rejected by Western doctors. But in a community that has a different ethical system altogether, would it be right for the doctor to deny women the right to practice this ritual which they believe plays a beneficial role in the mother's and baby's health? Would it be right for the doctor to remove this patient's autonomy for the sake of upholding non-maleficence...in other words, tearing one pillar down for the sake of another?

In the case of Haiti's cultural birthing practices, the priority for Western doctors lies in working with the local community to find the right balance between respecting the local customs and traditions while simultaneously offering Western medical advice. Prerna explains there are three major healing traditions in the world. "The US and most other Western countries practice Western biomedicine, which focuses on illness being caused by chemical imbalances in the body. The other two health practices are supernatural health practice and holistic health practice." She argues that cultural competency training and understanding of all three healing traditions are important to improving health outcomes and preventing mortality among patient populations who experience significantly different health realities.

We see examples of such differing health realities all the time. One patient at our clinic did not want to get the COVID-19 vaccine because she believed her grandmother's Russian ginger tea recipe would offer her safer protection than any vaccine. Another patient of ours who had uncontrolled Type 2 diabetes began taking a daily spoonful of cinnamon in place of her prescribed insulin because she "didn't like putting so many drugs in [her] body." My friend Titi remembers observing a patient who insisted on drinking a special green tea (his family's recipe) after his gastrointestinal surgery.

As Chaitanya Patel, the Internal Medicine resident who helped the Hindi patient with anemia in Chapter Three, shared with me: "What's important is being able to present the facts as well as understanding the patient's perspective. The analogy I've used multiple times is that it's better to attack from two different sides than just one. So, if they're going to use their [traditional healing] techniques, let us use our Western medicine techniques and we can take it on together. By giving them the motivation and confidence that we're doing this together, it's a mutual compromise rather than being an act of shutting them and their beliefs down."

This advice works well when the traditional practices are harmless and possibly have great health benefits as well. Our clinic's attending physician agreed to let our diabetic patient off the insulin and have her continue her daily cinnamon, as long as her blood glucose levels remained stable, and she came to her regular appointments so we could closely monitor her condition. But when patients adhere to cultural beliefs and traditional practices that cause more harm than good, how do providers navigate this? Such balance is possible only when there is a cultural broker, one who is both competent and experienced with working within these cultures, to bridge this gap.

* * *

Rob and Melodie Adams are what I would call "cross-cultural experts." Having lived in India for over ten years in cities and villages alike, Rob and Melodie have grown to cherish India as their second home and its people and culture like their own.

Now, they run a popular YouTube Channel called, "Chai and Coaching," which is a community of people that build bridges, provide information, and foster cross-cultural connections. The channel, which is targeted toward new immigrants in America (especially Indian immigrants), features topics ranging from apartment hunting to improving credit score to finding a job in the States, and discusses different challenges and solutions new immigrants might encounter in the US.

I got to chat with Rob and Melodie about their experiences with living in India. One of the greatest culture shocks they experienced there, as they shared with me, was the healthcare. Melodie's first child was born in India, at the Cloudnine Hospital in Bangalore to be precise. Cloudnine Hospitals is the number one pregnancy and maternity hospital chain in all of India. The founder, neonatologist Dr. R Kishore Kumar, had studied medicine in Australia and practiced abroad in the UK. Upon returning to India and seeing the miserable state of the crowded government hospitals and poorly managed private nursing centers, Dr. Kumar decided to found Cloudnine Hospitals with the hope of providing high quality care for expecting mothers and their newborns across the country.

Rob and Melodie were incredibly lucky to be able to receive their prenatal care at Cloudnine. Even though it was "super affordable compared to America," according to Rob, it was nevertheless *the* nicest hospital to have a baby in India.

One of the perks of this hospital was it offered antenatal coaching classes (referred to as prenatal classes in America). In these classes, expecting mothers and their families learned the basics about their baby's anatomy and physiology, planning their birth, breastfeeding, staying healthy during pregnancy, and more. The antenatal class was taught by Dr. Kumar himself, who stood at the front of a large room that seated a little less than one hundred people. Among these hundred people, Rob and Melodie were the only white people in the crowd. Almost all the patients who came to Cloudnine for care were well-to-do Bangaloreans who worked in tech, owned businesses, and came from the nice neighborhoods of the city. Many of the expecting mothers were there along with their family members: mostly husbands, a few mothers, and even fewer mothers-in-law.

As the audience came to a hush, Dr. Kumar asked through the microphone:

"Raise your hand if you have been taking saffron as a supplement."

Just about every expecting mother in the audience raised her hand, except Melodie. Rob and Melodie looked around in surprise. Dr. Kumar then pointed to a woman in the front row and asked her to share why.

"Because the saffron will help my baby have lighter skin," she shared.

A series of nods and hearty chuckles of acknowledgment filled the room. Dr. Kumar smiled and nodded.

"All right. Now, raise your hand if you have been taking your iron supplements."

This time, every expecting mother in the audience kept her hand down and shook her head no, except Melodie who raised her hand. When asked why not, one of the mothers who shook her head explained, "Iron will make my baby dark. That is why I'm not taking any iron." Everyone nodded emphatically, especially the mothers-in-law and older folks in the audience. Dr. Kumar nodded with acknowledgement, and then explained:

"If your husband has dark skin, your baby is going to have dark skin. Whether or not you take saffron or iron supplements will not determine the skin color of your baby."

Dr. Kumar went on to explain that skipping iron supplements could have a detrimental effect on the mother and baby. These families were largely vegetarian and ate no meat, which meant that iron deficiency was already a risk factor. To be skipping iron supplements on top of this vegetarian diet could push the mother into dangerous anemia.

Everyone laughed heartily in response to Dr. Kumar's comment. Many of these patients belonged to the younger generation that was more Western in their thinking. They understood Dr. Kumar's point that these preferences for saffron and avoidance of iron were no more than superstitious. However, there were still a large portion of mothers in the audience who lived in joint families with their mothers-in-law and other older relatives that still very much believed in these traditions. Odds were these mothers would continue to practice these traditional medicinal practices at home, either due to personal belief or due to elders in the family that would encourage or force them to follow these folk traditions.

"As a patient's doctor, you're not the only person they speak to every day to manage their health," Dr. Sulagna Roy, a Bangladeshi doctor in the UK, explains. "They wake up every day and make their choices based on their cultural upbringing." The role of family is a huge one in determining the health-related choices a patient makes, as was the case with these expecting mothers. In these cases, how do doctors factor in this cultural upbringing of the patient while also ensuring the patient gets the best care possible? How can they integrate Western medical practices with the cultural beliefs their patients hold?

Much of Western medicine is centered around the practice of evidence-based medicine (EBM). EBM ensures that providers administer treatments that have been extensively researched and studied under controlled conditions in order to maximize benefit and minimize harm for patients. As such, providers often face difficulty in permitting complementary and alternative medicines (CAM) that have not been studied under such controlled conditions. Part of the reason behind this difficulty is that providers don't know how these CAM treatments might interact with the body and with other medications.

For example, AIDS patients in the 1990s who used garlic for therapeutic purposes found that garlic's naturally occurring chemical compounds were adversely interacting with the patients' antiretroviral medications. A 2002 study featured in the *Journal of the American Medicine Association* (JAMA) found that garlic reduced levels of saquinavir (an antiretroviral medication for treating HIV) in the blood by up to 50 percent (Vastag, 2000). The biggest danger lies in believing things that are natural are also safe. While herbs and natural substances might be effective, they can also be incredibly potent and lead to herb-drug interactions with unknown and unintended consequences.

This is all the more reason for why we should prioritize funding research within the fields of integrative medicine and ethnopharmacology to study such substances. Two decades ago, over 25 percent of prescription medications had at least one plant or herb-derived substance among their ingredients, and this number has only grown since as more and more pharmaceutical companies develop plant-based medicines to treat illnesses (Duke, 1993). If we want patients and providers to start recognizing naturally occurring herbs and plants as potent substances, then we must work to produce research that places these natural remedies on the same level of potency as man-made drugs. Only then can herb-drug interactions be given the same level of attention as drug-drug interactions.

Yale pharmacology professor Yung-Chi Cheng is one such individual who has worked to pioneer this field of WE (Western-Eastern) medicine, which focuses on the blending of microscopic single-disease targets with traditional Chinese therapies. Through his research, Professor Cheng hopes to show the world how nutrition and herbal medicines of past traditions still hold immense value in today's world. "Chinese medicine works by taking advantage of multiple chemicals, but also the capability of different organs in metabolizing these chemicals," he explains.

Professor Cheng and his team developed a drug, called YIV-906, that shows a new way of treating liver cancer and hepatitis B with minimal side effects. The chemical formulation of their drug is based on traditional herbal medicines used for stomach ailments as described in ancient Chinese texts. According to a March 2020 Yale press release, Professor Cheng and his research partners have launched an international clinical trial for YIV-906 (the first ever clinical trial of such scale for a botanical drug) in over twenty institutions across the US, China, Taiwan, and Hong Kong (Belli, 2020). By using cultural healing traditions to inspire his search, Professor Cheng has pioneered a new path in the field of pharmacology and cancer research. "It's a totally new paradigm. I've been met with a lot of suspicion, but I think the results will speak for themselves."

Cultural healing traditions will continue to exist as long as the culture lives on and shunning or excluding such traditions from our practice of medicine is not conducive to achieving full health. As psychologist and professor Dr. Fayth Parks shares in her famous TEDx Talk: "Healing traditions are legitimate partners in conventional medicine and healing for those patients who are closely tied to their cultural identity. They can enlighten our modern quest to find pathways to greater well-being." The best way for the scientific community to work toward building harmony with these cultural practices is to start integrating these practices into our evidence-based medicine.

* * *

While achieving this sort of harmony can be difficult, it isn't impossible. When done right, it can make an incredible difference in the patient's life. In fact, I've seen this firsthand with my grandmother. I was in my senior year of high school when I learned that Ammamma (my maternal grandmother) suffered for over two decades from severe clinical depression and obsessive-compulsive disorder (OCD). I had no idea it ran in my family, matrilineally for generations. Mental illness was a topic that was rarely discussed. Whenever I used to ask Amma about her childhood, she would occasionally mention Ammamma was very sick and bedridden for many years. I had always assumed it was something related to her physical health.

It turned out Ammamma was bedridden because she mentally couldn't get herself to get out of bed. She was frequently overcome with *chikaaku,* which *very* roughly translates from Telugu as "irritation" or "anger" or "the sensation of feeling gross." If I had to describe it, *chikaaku* most resembles the feeling one gets when PMSing, except Ammamma's *chikaaku* wasn't limited to her periods. She would lash out unexpectedly at family members. She grew tired after even the simplest of tasks. She would wash her hands every time she touched something. She would spend hours at a time taking a bath. She was (and still is) an extreme germophobe (although now to less of an extreme). She rarely left the house because she lacked the motivation to do so (not to mention all the germs that would bring back that feeling of *chikaaku*). Tatayya (my grandfather) was always out of town on some business trip, and Ammamma was almost always in bed. This was in large part why Amma and both my aunts had to learn to take care of themselves at an early age.

Ammamma never knew this *chikaaku* was something she needed to get help for, nor did she know how to get help. She prayed multiple times a day to each of the different photos of *Ammoru* and *Venkateswara* and *Vinayaka* and *Krishna* and *Sai Baba* and *Shiva* and *Parvathi* that covered the walls of the house. She prayed to the point that she began seeing them every so often. *Ammoru* (the Mother Goddess) would often appear in front of Ammamma, dressed in a saffron-colored *pattu cheera* and large red *bottu* on her forehead. After all, Ammamma was *Ammoru's* namesake. Sometimes, *Ammoru* would tell her to take another shower or to stay inside the house. Other times *Ammoru* would help her, like the time she came and gave Ammamma a *kismis* (yellow raisin) packet when Tatayya went into hypoglycemia. To this day, I get chills when I listen to her talk about her miraculous encounters with *Ammoru*.

And yet, that was also the problem. *Ammoru* was the Mother Goddess. She was a Divine Being, and to be graced with her presence and guidance was a blessing. Why fix something that was a blessing? Ammamma never talks about why she waited for two decades to get treatment, but I suspect this might have been a part of it. It was only after many years, after seeing how her quality of life and her time with her now-grown-up children and young grandchildren was compromised, did she agree to seek proper treatment.

Upon the suggestion of a family friend, Ammamma went to see a psychiatrist in the city. Her doctor, who was actually a distant relative of ours, understood better than anyone the cultural fears and hesitations Ammamma carried. He understood why she was reluctant to begin treatment. He understood why she opted to use folk remedies and rituals in place of medication. And because he could understand where she was coming from, he was in the best position to help Ammamma find a balance between her health needs and cultural beliefs.

He prescribed a low dose of sertraline (an antidepressant medication that treats symptoms of both depression and OCD) in order to help Ammamma regain control of her life. But along with the sertraline, he assured her that she need not lose her relationship with *Ammoru* as a result. She could remain just as devotional, but would now have the mental energy and capability to make the most of her devotion. And sure enough, Ammamma showed incredible improvement. Once bedridden with *chikaaku*, she now keeps herself busy with household chores and conversations with family and her favorite TV serials. She always keeps her sertraline on hand, which she refers to as her *"kopam billalu"* or "anger pills." Needless to say, her doctor won her trust, and she has successfully adhered to her treatment regimen ever since.

A few summers ago, I had the opportunity to volunteer as a scribe at this doctor's psychiatry clinic in Vijayawada, India. While I thought Ammamma's situation was pretty bad, some of the patients I worked with at the clinic suffered from even more severe cases. I recall one patient who would bathe up to ten times per day because *"Ammoru cheppindhi.* The Goddess told [him] to." As was the case with Ammamma, his symptoms were not acknowledged as a sign of mental illness by his family. They sought the help of traditional healers, religious priests, and *tantriks* to alleviate their problems, not recognizing these problems were psychiatric in nature (at least according to Western medicine). The patient was soon diagnosed with co-morbid OCD and schizophrenia and was kept in the clinic for sessions of inpatient treatment and therapy.

There are many barriers that prevent individuals from seeking care in the first place, including problems of stigma, discrimination, distrust of urban professionals, religious beliefs, and mental health illiteracy (Kumar, 2012). Unless the symptoms are very severe, most people in the rural areas of India (like the patients who traveled for hours to get to the psychiatry clinic in Vijayawada) do not recognize their problems as mental illnesses. Rather, they believe their symptoms to be messages from God or possession by demons and evil spirits (Banerjee, 2015). In fact, one of my favorite movies growing up (a 2005 Tamil movie called *Chandramukhi*) delves into this clash between Western medical vs. Eastern spiritual approaches to mental illness. What the patient's psychiatrist deemed to be split-personality disorder as a manifestation of her childhood trauma, the family's priest deemed to be possession by an angry spirit. The crux of the movie's plot centers around how the psychiatrist and priest work together to treat the patient.

In Luhrmann's study of schizophrenia, one patient from Chennai reported hearing voices from *Hanuman*, the Hindu god of strength and bravery. *Hanuman* would play with her and tell her to do chores like cooking and cleaning (Lurhmann, 2015). In cases where the voices were more violent, people would travel for days and weeks to Hanumanthapuram, South India. The temple in Hanumanthapuram is devoted to the incarnation of the Hindu god *Shiva* (of whom *Hanuman* is an avatar), who is believed to purge evil spirits from the body (Kennedy, 2010).

The best way to address the problems that arise with cultural diversity is to ensure mental health care providers are familiar with the cultural norms in the geographical area where they are delivering treatment. They must adopt an ethno-specific and community-based approach to mental health care apart from the already existing medical and biological approaches. This way, treatment will be personalized for each individual and will be much more effective (Gopalkrishnan, 2015).

Currently, there are a very limited number of mental health care providers in India. Moreover, these providers are often not well-versed in the particular cultural nuances familiar to the patient. The provider might try to impose a medication or treatment plan that is not compatible with the patient's cultural background. This can create increased stress, reduce patient trust, and perhaps even worsen the patient's condition.

One plan India and several other countries in the Global South are currently working on is to train traditional healers in the proper treatment of mental illnesses. Patients from rural villages tend to have more faith in their local *shamans, tantriks, sangomas,* and other healers than they do in urban trained professionals, particularly because these healers are more familiar with the beliefs and customs these patients practice. Now with a growing immigrant population in the US, healthcare providers here have begun to adopt a similar approach in collaborating with community members and spiritual leaders to provide culturally-concordant care for their patients. By training and collaborating with such traditional healers, patients from these communities can receive proper care from those they trust, rather than having to go out of their comfort zone to receive treatment from professionals who do not understand their background and culture. This collaboration between traditional healers and medical practitioners is necessary for bridging the patient's cultural beliefs with their health needs.

CHAPTER 6

FIRST IMPRESSIONS

"If you can't see that your own culture has its own set of interests, emotions, and biases, how can you expect to deal successfully with someone else's culture?"

— ANNE FADIMAN, *THE SPIRIT CATCHES*
YOU AND YOU FALL DOWN

It was a bright sunny April Fool's morning, and our COVID vaccine clinic had been going unusually smoothly. Every patient arrived on time today (a rare occurrence), which meant there were enough rooms available for the fifteen-minute post-vaccination wait with no backup in patient flow. My coworker and I were tag-teaming with escorting patients between the vaccination room and waiting rooms, checking patients in and out on the computer, and wiping rooms clean between visits.

One of the challenging parts of coordinating patient flow during vaccine clinic is assigning rooms to patients to wait their fifteen minutes post-vaccination. Because a majority of patients were still receiving their first dose at this time, it was imperative that our patients maintained distance between each other. To ensure social distancing, we made sure to seat each patient in their own waiting room. There were some instances when couples would arrive together to get vaccinated, in which case we would have them sit together in Room One (the only room with two patient chairs) in order to have more waiting rooms open for other patients.

Two elderly Chinese patients, Mr. and Mrs. Li, checked in at the front desk at around 10:20 a.m., as indicated by the green "Checked In" text next to their names on the computer. I walked to the lobby and found them sitting together in the two chairs next to the window. After confirming with the receptionist at the front desk that they came together, I called out their names and asked them to follow me to the vaccination room.

Mrs. Li walked with great vigor and a pep in her step, keeping up with my relatively fast pace. Mr. Li, on the other hand, walked very slowly and hesitantly behind us. Mrs. Li walked into the vaccination room, sat down, and pulled up her sleeve. I motioned for Mr. Li to also take a seat in the room so he could wait with her, but he shook his head. After a few failed attempts of asking him to wait inside, I took him to Room One to wait until Mrs. Li was done.

I heard the beep of Mrs. Li's timer, which meant she was done getting the vaccine and that the fifteen-minute countdown had begun. I brought Mrs. Li to Room One and took Mr. Li to the vaccination room. After Mr. Li was done and his timer began counting down, I brought him back to Room One to spend the wait with Mrs. Li. I asked both of them if they would like any water to drink. They shook their heads no.

After fifteen minutes, Mrs. Li's timer began to beep loudly. I stepped in and took the timer from Mrs. Li as she began to get up from her chair.

"It's okay, you can stay here if you'd like!" I quickly interrupted.

Mrs. Li looked confused. "No thanks, I will leave."

"Don't you want to wait with your husband?" I asked.

Her eyes widened with shock, and she began to shake her head vigorously.

"No, no, no, he's not my husband. I don't know him!"

Oh my god. My jaw dropped. I looked at Mr. Li sitting next to her. He was staring at the wall with a blank expression, not even looking up at me or Mrs. Li. I could feel my cheeks flushing with embarrassment.

Mrs. Li waved goodbye to me and proceeded to head out. Mr. Li followed suit shortly after. Though Mrs. Li didn't seem to think anything of the mix-up, I on the other hand was absolutely mortified. I had mistakenly assumed Mr. and Mrs. Li were a married couple simply because they were both elderly, shared the same Chinese last name, and happened to be sitting next to each other in the waiting room. What was worse was I wasn't the only one who made this assumption. I guess the front desk must have also made the same mistake in informing us they were here together, because they saw Mr. and Mrs. Li arrive at the clinic at the same time.

Why didn't I just *ask* them if they were together, instead of assuming they were? I had checked with the front desk, but I didn't make the effort to check with the patients directly. Though Mr. Li spoke no English, Mrs. Li spoke a few words of English and seemed to understand me quite well. I could have double checked with her. At the very least, I could have taken a hint based on how Mr. Li was hesitating to enter the vaccination room with Mrs. Li despite my multiple attempts to get him inside.

I wonder how this situation would have played out differently had I been less ignorant of these cues, had I been less hasty to make assumptions, had I paid more attention. Would I have made the same assumption if this was an elderly Indian couple?

In the grand scheme of things, my ignorance and presumptive biases likely had little effect on the care Mr. Li and Mrs. Li received. They both got their vaccines, and they both seemed pretty unperturbed by my mishap. But still, it is unwise to assume such biases and assumptions won't lead to more serious repercussions in the future. What exactly might these consequences be when such biases are left unchecked, and whose responsibility is it to keep these biases in check?

* * *

Jacqueline Melecio, the daughter of Dominican immigrants in the US, has devoted her life's work to studying such topics related to cultural diversity, equity, and bias. Her PhD dissertation was about the integration of cultural competency in the delivery of mental health services to Latinos. Now, she is the CEO of Equity Dynamics, a consulting firm focused on addressing and strengthening the corporate understanding of race, culture, and diversity within complex systems of care. "I'm interested in looking not only at the individual perspective, but also at the organizational support for cultural competency and thinking about what needs to be in place in order for it to work," shared Jacqueline.

Back in the day, Jacqueline used to work as a Spanish interpreter in the interpretation and translation services department of a human services organization that addressed housing, education, healthcare, legal assistance, and basically every type of human service you could think of. One day she would be at the doctor's office interpreting for a patient, and the next day she would be at the courthouse interpreting for a client.

There was one particular instance in which she was interpreting for a social worker doing a foster adoption case. The social worker was visiting a couple's home to do an assessment and determine whether it was safe for the foster child to be adopted into this family. Jacqueline went along with her to help with interpretation for the visit, since the couple only spoke Spanish.

The wife welcomed Jacqueline and the social worker into the house. As they followed the wife inside, Jacqueline couldn't help but smile. The house reminded her a lot of her childhood home. The warm scent of plantain soup cooking on the stove, the photos of saints on the walls, even the flower-patterned porcelain-ware sitting on the table—these were the classic signs of a proper Dominican household.

The wife led them to the living room, where they all took a seat. Her kids all rushed into the living room, hoping to catch bits and pieces of the conversation about the adoption of their potential new brother. The wife was kind and genial, answering the social worker's questions and posing questions of her own. Though she was slightly anxious about the whole process, she was eagerly and actively participating in the conversation.

A few minutes later, the husband entered the room, and the wife suddenly became quiet. The husband began to answer the questions, even though some of these questions were part of an ongoing conversation between the wife and the social worker. The social worker made direct eye contact with the wife as she asked questions, but the wife simply looked at her husband and he answered in her place. A couple of times, the husband paused and looked at his wife, at which point she spoke up and answered the question. But for the most part, the husband did the majority of the talking. This back-and-forth between the husband and social worker continued for the rest of the conversation as his wife and children listened quietly.

After about a half hour of interviewing, the social worker and Jacqueline thanked the couple for their time and hospitality and left the house. On their way back to the office, the social worker expressed her concerns with Jacqueline.

"This seemed like a spousal abuse situation of some kind. The wife was sweet, but I'm worried about her husband."

As part of the assessments, the human services team uses their experience and skills to pick up nonverbal cues beyond just the verbal conversation with the family. The social worker noticed the wife fell silent when her husband entered the room and presumed the husband was intimidating or threatening the wife into not speaking. If the parents were suspected to have an abusive relationship, it would mean the child would not be adopted into their family.

Jacqueline understood why the social worker might have assumed there to be abuse, but there was another component of this interaction that hadn't been considered.

"It might have been a cultural thing," Jacqueline clarified. "In Dominican families, the husband is usually in charge of the household. So, when he comes into the room, it's often the wife's way of showing respect to him."

As a child of Dominican immigrants, Jacqueline grew up in a similar cultural environment as this family, so she understood the unspoken dynamic of this couple.

"It's not abuse because notice how the wife *did* participate as the conversation went on," Jacqueline pointed out.

The wife indeed participated when the husband yielded the conversation to her, or when he paused and looked at her to continue. Because this was a familiar dynamic to Jacqueline as occurred frequently in her own family, she was able to look past the immediate first impression of abusive behavior. It wasn't that the husband was abusing her. Rather, it was that the wife saw it as a way of paying respect to her husband by letting him speak first.

Thankfully upon further investigation and a second visit to the family's home, there was no sign of abuse to be determined. The social worker was right to look into the nonverbal cues as a part of her assessment for red flags. But because she failed to take the cultural components into account, she ended up drawing the wrong conclusion from those cues. The social worker misinterpreted the wife's deference and cultural respect to her husband as a red flag because of her unfamiliarity with family and power dynamics in Dominican culture. Fortunately, Jacqueline was there to shed light on that cultural component of the interaction and rule out the possibility of suspected abuse in the family. And in the end, the foster child was successfully adopted into the family.

In this situation, the responsibility of countering the biases and judgments of the social worker fell to Jacqueline. As someone who also shared a similar cultural heritage and upbringing as this family, Jacqueline was familiar and competent with the typical family dynamics of the culture.

However, cultural competency isn't always enough. In fact, when used on its own, cultural competency can lead to adverse consequences. The term "competency" exudes a sense of being all-knowing and all-powerful, which can create an unhealthy power dynamic. More importantly, the term implies that one has learned everything they need to learn about a certain culture or group of people, when in fact learning is a never-ending process. It is this false security of knowledge that can lead to the formation of biases and stereotypes, where one makes a judgment about someone by virtue of the cultural group to which they belong.

We see examples of cultural stereotyping and implicit bias all too often in healthcare. A nurse who has taken a course in cross-cultural training fails to treat a Hispanic patient's postoperative pain because "[she] 'knows' that Hispanic patients over-express the pain they are feeling" (Tervalon & Murray-Garcia, 1998). A doctor fails to acknowledge a Jewish patient's request for a follow-up appointment because she remembers reading "Jews can be extra vocal and demanding of assistance." A Muslim provider dismisses a Muslim patient's symptoms as due to Ramadan fasting, when the patient has actually refrained from fasting due to her preexisting symptoms. When providers make clinical decisions based solely on their "self-proclaimed cultural expertise" rather than the individual circumstances of their patients, the health of their patients can be compromised. In fact, a 2017 nursing textbook was pulled by its publisher due to its inclusion of such dangerously presumptive and overly simplistic portrayals and stereotypes of various cultures (Sini, 2017).

This is why cultural humility is a far more desirable goal for cultural brokers and healthcare providers (for anyone in fact) than is cultural competency. While cultural competency is a topic or subject that people feel must be learned and mastered, cultural humility is a philosophy, a mindset one uses to handle different situations in unique ways. When one looks beyond culture, race, and ethnicity, each of us is a complicated multidimensional human being with our own histories & stories. Cultural humility recognizes this uniqueness and understands no individual can learn and know everything there is to know about any given culture or group of people. This humility is what enables us to be open to learning new things and shifting our existing knowledge base. As Melanie Tervalon, one of the first researchers to coin this term, explains it: "Cultural humility challenges us to think more deeply about what culture is and how it doesn't mean thinking about a list of traits that you can ascribe to people." This focus on lifelong learning and self-improvement is the key to dispelling stereotypes and biases.

In Jacqueline's case, she was not only knowledgeable of the culture to look past the first impression of abuse, but she was also humble enough to understand that abuse could still be a valid possibility. She didn't make a decision based solely upon her knowledge of the culture, even if it was her own culture. She understood that even within a given culture, people can hold different views and follow different practices. By pursuing a second visit to the family's home as opposed to writing off the possibility of abuse solely based on cultural practices, Jacqueline was able to ensure a safe and loving family environment for the adopted son. Her delicate balance of cultural competency and cultural humility is what allows her to serve as a successful cultural broker.

* * *

Prithvi Mavuri, the Internal Medicine resident who took care of the elderly Telugu father in Chapter Two, sees cultural humility as the single most important factor in establishing rapport and preventing stereotypes when working with patients of different cultures. "The guesswork is taken out when you spend the time and talk to them," he explained. "And when you seek out that information and learn more about where they are coming from, you'll get that perspective."

Unfortunately, not all providers prioritize this aspect of cultural humility in their care of patients. A patient of Prithvi's fellow resident (let's call her Maria) was in the ICU because she had been showing severe symptoms. A week earlier, Maria had developed a dry cough and fever. Though her daughter was worried, Maria thought nothing of it. It was normal to try to heal at home using herbal remedies before resorting to an expensive hospital visit.

Maria spent the next few days using her *abuela's* (grandmother's) remedies. When Maria was younger and suffered frequently from cough and sore throat, her *abuela* would take dried *gordolobo*, a flowering plant commonly found in Central and Northern Mexico, and infuse it into hot water to make an herbal tea. *Gordolobo* was used for centuries to cure colds, flu symptoms, pneumonia, bronchitis, and other respiratory issues (Rittenhouse, 2019). Maria was positive that her *gordolobo* tea would help her recover from these symptoms.

Unfortunately, her condition worsened. About a week from the onset of her symptoms, no longer able to bear the pain and fatigue, she decided to go to the hospital. Maria was immediately brought into the ICU and roomed in the isolation unit. Everyone who entered her room, from the nurses to the technicians to the doctors, was decked head to toe in their isolation gowns and face shields and other protective gear.

Maria looked confusedly at the hubbub around her. She spoke only Spanish, so she wasn't able to understand what the doctors and nurses around her were saying. All she could fathom from the bustling bodies and overlapping voices in the isolation room was she was diagnosed with COVID-19.

Because Maria was placed in the COVID isolation unit, her daughter wasn't allowed to enter due to safety and exposure concerns. The daughter couldn't be there in person to explain to Maria what was going on, so she coordinated with one of the nurses on the floor to set up a video conference call in order to speak with her mother and translate for her.

Maria stayed in the isolation unit for several weeks, continuing to receive oxygen and remdesivir (an antiviral medication for treating COVID). She had developed a few complications along the way, including a bacterial infection that affected her lungs and breathing, but she slowly began to show signs of improvement.

A few weeks later, the resident responsible for Maria's care came back in to check on her.

"Hi Maria, how are you feeling now?" the resident asked.

"*Hola mama. El doctor esta preguntando como se siente ahora,*" Maria's daughter translated through video call on the iPad. "The doctor is asking how you're feeling now."

Maria smiled weakly. "*Me siento mejor que esta manana pero estoy muy cansada.* I'm feeling better than this morning. I'm just very tired."

The resident spoke with Maria for a few minutes longer to assess her condition, and Maria's daughter translated. Maria refused to take any steroids or opiates for her pain. She insisted she was fine and her pain would go away on its own course. After deciding Maria had sufficiently recovered, the resident sent Maria home with some oxygen and antibiotics for treatment of any residual symptoms and her bacterial infection.

Later that day during lunch break, the resident chatted with Prithvi and the other residents about the case.

"I can't believe she thought drinking that tea would help her get cured from COVID," the resident shared in disbelief.

Another resident chimed in. "That's so crazy that she took so long to come into the hospital. How did she think she was going to be okay?"

The first resident shrugged. "No idea."

Prithvi remembered feeling appalled as he watched this conversation happen. If his grandmother were in Maria's situation, she would have done the same thing. Prithvi, coming from a Telugu Hindu family whose cultural and religious identity was closely intertwined with their healing practices, understood the role these healing traditions played in their care. When his grandmother got sick, she often made a *kashayam* (herbal tea) to cure her sore throat and shortness of breath, much like Maria's *gordolobo* tea.

Prithvi couldn't help but wonder, "Would my grandmother receive the same disdain from my colleagues if she were the one to come into the ICU? Would her cultural beliefs and practices be brushed aside just as quickly?" Prithvi grew up surrounded by these cultural traditions, and so he resonated more deeply with Maria's story than his fellow residents who were only ever exposed to Western allopathic medicine. He took the time to empathize with Maria and understand the reason behind her decision to delay hospital care.

Interestingly enough, Prithvi's story reminded me of a conversation I had with my editor when writing the initial drafts of this book. As they were reading the very first story in this book (about the Vietnamese family who performed *cao gio* coining on their child in Chapter One), they confessed to me, "I'll admit to a cultural bias. When I read the intention of coining, my immediate thought was *'That's silly, it doesn't work like that.'* Then I realized that that's how the insensitive doctors think! It doesn't matter what I, a doctor, or anyone else thinks of a practice that isn't harmful. It isn't our place to judge, and cultural brokers are an important part of defining what is culture and what is a situation that requires intervention."

While healthcare providers do indeed have a responsibility to guide the patient toward better health, they have an equally important responsibility to respect and accommodate the patient's own beliefs without presenting bias of their own. It is not their place to judge the patient's beliefs, as Prithvi's colleagues had done. As Prithvi often says, "Treatment is not just limited to the medical therapy you provide. It includes how you speak to them and how you connect with them."

And when providers fail to respect and accommodate their patient's beliefs, the burden falls upon cultural brokers like Prithvi to step in and counter the assumptions and judgments made by providers. Through the practice of cultural humility, cultural brokers act as agents of change in the healthcare setting and beyond. They counter the biases (both implicit and explicit) held by others on the provider team and ensure the patient's culture is represented in the most honest and authentic way.

CHAPTER 7

THE ART OF TEACHING

"Education is not the learning of facts, but the training of minds to think."

— ALBERT EINSTEIN

Dr. Hla Thein grew up in Burma, where he was taught by monks for most of his early education. He later attended medical school in Rangoon, then moved to Thailand to work for the United Nations where he provided medical care to Khmer Rouge refugees. Eventually, Dr. Thein settled in Fiji, where he lived for eighteen years with his theologian wife, Florence, and his pro-golfer son, Ederil.

However, this peaceful life in Fiji wasn't enough for Dr. Thein. He wanted a challenge. So, he decided to move to Pukapuka, a small isolated three-square-kilometer-wide part of the Cook Islands, to focus on the treatment of chronic conditions among Pacific Islander populations.

There had not been a doctor in Pukapuka since 2005. Doctors signed two-year contracts to stay on the island and provide care for the 450 people who lived there, but many of them would break their contracts early. Pukapuka was notorious for its boredom, isolation, language barriers, and difficulty of disease management. Naturally, no one wanted to be the doctor there. Other doctors would even try to discourage Dr. Thein from taking the position. He didn't heed their warnings. He wanted a challenge, and this seemed like the perfect one.

The islanders of Pukapuka traditionally followed a healthy diet that included taro, crab, fish, pumpkin, and other locally sourced foods. But over time, the islanders grew to develop an unhealthy dependence on canned, processed, and fast foods. As clinical psychologist and local islander Amelia Hokule'a Borofsky inquires in her *Atlantic* article, "How do you get a Pacific Islander who, thanks to WWII, loves canned corned beef, Spam, and rice, to start eating arugula?"

This was precisely the question that had stumped every doctor who had previously been in Pukapuka. How were they supposed to treat the islanders' hypertension, obesity, and diabetes if they could not even convince the islanders to change their eating habits?

Dr. Thein understood early on that his patients would not heed his words if he simply educated them with facts and science. Facts meant nothing to these islanders whose eating habits had become entrenched in their daily lives. In fact, studies have shown that mere knowledge does not produce behavioral change, especially in the early stages of intervention. While people may know the facts, they exempt themselves from the consequences because of their tendency to believe they are the exception to the norm (Raynor, 2007).

So, Dr. Thein decided to use two different techniques:

1. Teaching by example
2. Shaming

Dr. Thein began by growing a huge vegetable garden in his home, growing all kinds of produce like lettuce, tomatoes, cucumbers, garlic, radishes, *bok choy*, and *rukau*. He even enlisted the help of his hospital staff in tending the garden during hospital work hours. At first, everyone was confused by why he was having his nurses pull weeds in the garden instead of drawing blood in the hospital. But slowly, the villagers began to gather around to watch Dr. Thein and the hospital staff tend the garden. They wanted a garden like his in their own homes, and so they began to send children to ask Dr. Thein for vegetable seeds. Within months, every family on the island had their own vegetable garden.

At the end of the year, Dr. Thein arranged for an island-wide feast. The only rules were the food had to be made entirely from locally sourced items like coconut crab and taro, and the village leaders had to organize the entire event from preparing the food to presenting the feast. The feast was a huge success. It was a seminal moment for the islanders in realizing that their own local foods were both delicious *and* healthy.

Now that Dr. Thein's technique of teaching by example had created a mental awareness and proclivity toward change among the islanders, the next step was to get them to make that change in their behavior. To do this, Dr. Thein employed shame. He would call out parents who fed their children instant noodles instead of baked *uto* (sprouted coconut) by posting it on the local government notice board for everyone to see...and laugh at. He often told his patients in his usual cheeky manner, "There is something wrong in a place where the parents are so fat and the children so skinny." Soon enough, every parent began to cook their child's lunch at home instead of sending them to school with processed and canned foods. This was an important step not just for the children's health, but also for the parents, who began eating the same healthy food they cooked for their children.

He used these techniques of shaming and joking not just with obesity and diabetes, but with all health-related concerns. Whenever a married man came into his clinic with an STD, Dr. Thein would not treat the man until he brought every single one of his sexual partners with him to the clinic for treatment. As embarrassing as it was for the man, Dr. Thein's shame tactic ensured the spread of these STDs was stopped in its tracks.

Dr. Thein's techniques, by Western standards, are horrific. The idea of publicly shaming one's patients to get them to change their lifestyle is one that would face immense pushback (and perhaps even lawsuits) in America. But this wasn't America, and these patients weren't Western in their thinking. Dr. Thein had spent the majority of his life living in Pacific Island communities and working with Islander populations. He never attended lectures on cross-cultural communication or seminars on diversity training, nor did he have to. He knew the culture based on his own life and personal experiences, and he had a thorough understanding of what would work with this community and what wouldn't.

The fact of the matter is that knowledge alone is not enough to create lasting behavioral change, and Dr. Thein understood this. If facts were enough on their own, then no one would eat McDonalds or smoke or skip their daily exercise ever again. The mere statistics of cancer- and obesity-related deaths would suffice in dropping cigarette and Big Mac sales. But unfortunately, simply telling a smoker that smoking is bad for them is not enough to incite change. Perhaps the patient knows that smoking causes cancer, but they can't get themselves to stop because they get really bad headaches without it and can't afford treatment. Or maybe the patient understands that smoking increases their risk of cardiovascular disease, but he can't seem to get away from it because all his friends smoke and he'll risk being shunned if he doesn't participate. Simply narrating the facts doesn't do any good when the underlying reasons for lack of behavioral change are left unaddressed. And more often than not, these underlying reasons are linked to the culture the patient is surrounded by.

* * *

A little over fifteen years ago, Tamara Katz used to serve as a volunteer at our clinic. Though she passed away in 2004 at the age of ninety, she is remembered to this day by our clinic staff for her candid personality and the meaningful impact she had on our Russian patients. It wasn't until I read her obituary and learned of her story as a Holocaust survivor that I realized the pain and hardship that had hid behind her vivid demeanor.

Born in 1914 as Tamara Kaplinski in Lida, Poland, she learned many languages at a young age, including Polish, Russian, German, Yiddish, and Hebrew. Her language skills would prove invaluable with helping translate for the many Russian patients at our clinic. In 1937, Tamara married a fellow Pole, Abraham Dworzinski, and in 1939, they had their first son Nathan (Wall, 2004).

Two years later, the Holocaust began. Her parents and husband were shot in a mass killing of Polish Jews, leaving her widowed with her three-year-old son. Tamara always kept a few blades of grass from the mass killing site in her handkerchief as a reminder to herself to make it out at all costs.

Tamara and her son spent the next several years on the run. She was able to pass as non-Jewish because of her bright blue eyes and fluent Polish. In 1944, she met and married Abraham Katz, a fellow refugee. By the end of the war a year later, Tamara and Abraham found themselves in a displaced persons camp in Austria, where they gave birth to their daughter Ruth. Finally, the family decided to escape from it all and moved to the United States in 1951, settling in San Francisco.

Her husband passed away a few years later due to a kidney condition that began during the war. Though widowed and alone in a new country, Tamara let nothing get to her. Instead, she decided to live her dream as a bookkeeper, eventually learning the business well enough that she opened her own antiques shop. Tamara was known among family and friends for her fiercely independent attitude. "That was her greatest strength, but it was also her greatest demise, too, as she got older," her daughter Ruth shared. "She thought she could still do things; she would forget that she wasn't fifty anymore."

In a way, her independent and autonomous mindset came directly out of her early life experiences. She was at death's doorstep and managed to escape. She worked incredibly hard to get to where she got to be, and she suffered many losses along the way. Perhaps that was why she would not tolerate it when others didn't similarly work for what they wanted, especially fellow Eastern Europeans.

Tamara began volunteering as a Russian interpreter at our clinic in the early 2000s. Many of our clinic's patients back then were elderly Russian folks who moved to San Francisco right after the Cold War. In fact, the neighborhood surrounding our clinic had (and still has) a prominent Russian community. Living in a majority-Russian neighborhood was associated with greater retention of Russian identity and lower rates of acculturation for Russian immigrants in the US (Miller, 2009). And sure enough, this was the case with our clinic's Russian patients. Be it in the bread lines or soup kitchen queues back in Russia, they were used to fighting for their demands. If they fought hard enough, they got what they wanted. This was what worked in Soviet Russia, so patients began to use the same approach here in the clinic. They came in with exceedingly unreasonable demands, hounding the front desk staff, nurses, and doctors incessantly until their demands were met.

Tamara was fed up with their behavior. Our clinic at the time was incredibly small with limited resources, yet the doctors and staff took on any and every burden in order to provide free medical care to our uninsured patients. Tamara wanted to make a point to these patients that their lack of gratitude and unruly behavior was intolerable.

"This is America," she told them. "You need to work for what you want. You can't just make demands."

Because she was much older than any of the patients, they looked up to her. "Go to school. Learn the language," she told them. "Do what you need to do, but don't just ask for things without working for them." Tamara not only helped the patients adjust their behavior, but she unknowingly inspired many of them to go out and get jobs and learn English. She might not have made the same impact if she was an outsider lecturing these patients about how important it was to learn English, or if she lacked familiarity with the unique cultural challenges these Russian patients faced in emigrating to and living in the US. But because the community saw how she led by example and regarded her as one of them, Tamara was able to encourage meaningful change among our clinic's Russian population. She transformed the community from within.

In fact, this is precisely the phenomenon we have been seeing with COVID vaccination efforts in the US, where members of the community have stepped up to inspire impactful change and lead by example. Every Sunday morning, Reverend Gabriel Salguero leads church service at The Gathering Place, an evangelical church in Orlando, Florida. He draws inspiration from biblical scriptures to preach his sermons to his largely Hispanic congregation, sometimes on expository topics like community and faith, other times on more textual topics like fasting and the Holy Spirit. One Sunday in March of 2021, Rev. Salguero decided to focus his sermon on a timelier topic: the COVID-19 vaccine. "In getting yourself vaccinated, you are helping your neighbor," he preached to his 300-member congregation. "God wants you to be whole so you can care for your community. So, think of vaccines as part of God's plan" (Hoffman, 2021).

Rev. Salguero is just one of thousands of cultural and religious leaders from a variety of faith backgrounds who have been working hard to encourage their communities to get vaccinated against COVID-19. By weaving together science and faith in their sermons, cultural leaders like Rev. Salguero have been able to use their positions of trust and leadership to serve as cultural brokers between the religious beliefs and health needs of their community. "There's just an avalanche of misinformation and maybe fear and anxiety that feeds that," Rev. Salguero acknowledges. "Our commitment is not to tell people what to do, but to make the information easily accessible and to give trustworthy platforms."

Cultural challenges have played a large role in vaccine hesitancy among minority communities, particularly during the early months of 2021. With both information and misinformation spread alike, it has been close to impossible for people to know what to believe, especially when some of these myths carry extreme cultural significance. Dr. Priya Jaisinghani, a board-certified Internal Medicine physician and current Endocrinology fellow at New York Presbyterian Weill Cornell, has spent the past year working to understand the reasons behind why vaccine rollout in the US has been so slow. Over the course of this quality improvement project, Dr. Jaisinghani and her team were surprised to find over 200 reasons for why people were hesitating to get vaccinated, even among minority communities. Some of these reasons included historical exploitation and mistrust among communities of color, belief in the protective qualities of home remedies (e.g., *gordolobo* tea & *kashayam/kaadha* tea), unsubstantiated claims of vaccine side-effects, or refusal of vaccination due to religious beliefs. For example, the United States Conference of Catholic Bishops stated in the spring of 2021, that Catholics should avoid receiving the Johnson & Johnson vaccine because it was developed using cell lines from an aborted fetus and therefore was "morally compromised and unacceptable" (Weise, 2021).

In cases like these, religious leaders and clergymen like Rev. Salguero are vital to addressing these concerns and countering these claims by using both scientific reasoning and moral judgment alike. In response to the statement made at the Conference of Catholic Bishops, Pope Francis declared the COVID-19 vaccine to be "morally acceptable" because of the grave danger the pandemic posed to the public and the distance of connection to the aborted fetus. Though the Vatican and US Conference of Catholic Bishops have stated that Johnson & Johnson vaccines should be avoided in favor of Pfizer or Moderna if possible, the Pope has made it clear that Catholics have a duty to protect both themselves and their neighbors by receiving the vaccine. If they choose to not be vaccinated, then they are morally obligated to wear a mask and maintain social distancing (Hoffman, 2021).

Members of the clergy are working to address these fears and hesitancies by providing both the facts and the necessary moral support toward choosing the vaccine. Some leaders have even offered their sacred spaces as vaccination sites in order to make the experience more comfortable for the members of their community. One prominent Sikh temple, Gurdwara Sahib of Fremont, served as a prominent vaccination site for the Bay Area's Desi community, including many of my friends and acquaintances. The outdoor vaccination tents and rows of distanced chairs not only streamlined the vaccination process, but also provided an opportunity for community members to connect with one another after many months of isolation.

Meanwhile on the opposite coast, a local BAPS (sect of Hinduism originating in Gujarat, India) chapter in Raleigh, partnered with Avance Care Pharmacy to organize a COVID-19 vaccination drive and provide vaccine education for their Indian patients. With the help of medical staff, volunteers, and other providers, BAPS Charities created a video with Gujarati subtitles to provide important information about the vaccine, featuring doctors and researchers from within the BAPS community. "BAPS Charities is a very well-known and reputable charity organization in the community," said Ritesh Patel, CEO of Avance Care Pharmacy. "When BAPS Charities offered an opportunity for a vaccination drive, we were excited about the collaboration. It's a privilege for Avance Care Pharmacy to partner with BAPS Charities for this vaccination drive."

Language plays an important role in conveying accurate information and building trust with the community, as BAPS Charities understood and skillfully implemented. Similarly, Imam Sheikh Salahadin Wazir, the founder and CEO of African and Immigrant Communities in America and local Muslim leader, worked with the International Rescue Committee (IRC) in Atlanta to create multilingual informational videos about the vaccine. Imam Wazir, who speaks over six different languages (including English, Amharic, Arabic, Harari, Oromo, and Somali) has played a vital role in encouraging vaccine acceptance among Muslim communities in the South (NRC-RIM, 2021).

In creating these videos with Imam Wazir, the IRC found that following these guidelines leads to the greatest success in reaching a wide audience. First, a cultural broker is chosen, usually a faith leader like Imam Wazir who is locally based and trusted by the community, to serve as the voice of the video. Next, the cultural broker makes a statement recognizing how COVID-19 poses a grave problem for their local community (e.g., "COVID-19 has caused much pain and suffering for our Muslim community in Atlanta") and express a desire to combat this problem together as a community. This bolsters a feeling of togetherness and provides encouragement to act in accordance with broader community interests.

Then, the broker acknowledges that while many myths and rumors about the vaccine do exist, they are false and baseless. By using both scientific proof (e.g., "The COVID-19 vaccine contains no animal products and is halal") and support from religious texts (e.g., "A verse in the Quran states that if you save one life, it is as if you have saved the life of all humanity"), these videos are able to directly address common community concerns. Finally, after filming and production, the videos are shared widely throughout the community. Imam Wazir and Atlanta's IRC uploaded the six multi-language videos to their respective pages on Facebook, Instagram, and YouTube. Additionally, Imam Wazir circulated the videos to his many community contacts via WhatsApp.

While many cultural brokers like Imam Wazir and Rev. Salguero fill formal roles in their community as religious leaders and members of their clergy, not all cultural brokers are so formally designated. In fact, many individuals have stepped up to serve informally as cultural brokers for their communities during the pandemic.

One of the challenges with the pandemic has been the difficulty in locating and removing the many sources of false information on the internet. There are thousands of fake news sources in English alone. Now add another language into the mix, and the task becomes close to impossible. To combat this issue, Dr. Tung Nguyen, an Internal Medicine specialist at UCSF, recently launched a website (VietCovid.org) to disseminate accurate vaccine information in Vietnamese (Bandlamudi, 2021). "Many younger Vietnamese Americans with a limited grasp of medical vocabulary in Vietnamese face a credibility gap speaking to their elders," Dr. Nguyen explains. "The younger people may know the science, but they can't explain it in a way that actually makes them credible in Vietnamese. Of course, if they do it in English, the older people won't know or care."

Dr. Nguyen's goal is to encourage and empower younger Vietnamese Americans to push back against these sources of misinformation and "speak with authority to their elders about the vaccine." With the help of his website, a large number of youths have stepped up to the plate to address these issues. In Southern California, a group of volunteers translates COVID-19 related news articles from English to Vietnamese. In Connecticut, a young man created an Instagram account (Viet Fake News Buster) to pinpoint and flag YouTube videos that carry false information. In the South Bay, the Vietnamese Round Table sends details to the local community about shelter-in-place guidelines and vaccination alerts (all in Vietnamese). "We've grown up being cultural brokers, informational brokers for our families," shares Vietnamese American Roundtable Secretary Christina Johnson.

"Now we're really utilizing that skill and expanding it to do it for our communities."

In a similar vein, Dr. Jaisinghani, being a first-generation Indian American physician, has also embraced her dual identity and unique role as a healthcare provider and cultural broker for her patients. In March of 2021, a second wave of the pandemic began to spread across India, killing hundreds of people within days and infecting thousands more. I remember being shocked at how every single one of my Indian friends had at least one relative that had passed away during the second wave. There were millions of people who were scrambling to find answers, but had no one to turn to.

It was at this time that a new app, Clubhouse, was launched on iOS. Clubhouse is an audio-based platform which connects individuals from around the world to participate in discussion rooms, providing a means of disseminating information about various topics and collaborating across borders. In fact, the first time I met Dr. Jaisinghani was in a Clubhouse room about how the COVID-19 pandemic was affecting mental health among South Asians. We saw hundreds of Indians and Indian Americans who came to Clubhouse in search of help amidst the chaos of the deadly second wave.

It was then that Dr. Jaisinghani, who up until that point had been serving as a Clubhouse panelist to moderate discussions about the COVID-19 crisis, stepped up to help these individuals who had nowhere else to turn to. She joined forces with a civilian group based in India through WhatsApp to make herself accessible for providing best practice guidelines and support for folks across the world. Alongside her work as an Endocrinology fellow, she would volunteer day and night with civilians in India to help them navigate the challenges of the pandemic, all through WhatsApp. "COVID-19 has been an extremely humbling time for us in our professional careers as physicians, but even more so personally as humans," Dr. Jaisinghani shares. "The disease which divided and distanced us from each other also brought us together as global citizens."

Even though cultural brokers like Dr. Jaisinghani, Tamara Katz, and Dr. Thein do educate their communities with facts to dispel myths and misinformation, they understand that it's not the facts that make the difference. The reason behind these cultural brokers' success comes from their shared sense of identity with their community. Their community sees the broker as "one of them." They acknowledge that these brokers have gotten to know and understand their community. Importantly, they respect that these brokers have stepped up to serve as role models and teach by example. This is what allows complete trust to take place and for meaningful change to happen.

CHAPTER 8

THE CONSTANT
OF CHANGE

"The art of life lies in a constant readjustment to our surroundings."

— KAKUZO OKAKURA, *THE BOOK OF TEA*

Pellegrino Riccardi is no stranger to navigating cultures. Pellegrino's name means, "pilgrim." It was as if his name had destined him for his life to come. As he shared in his TEDx talk, "My parents must have thought to themselves, 'Let's give him the name *pilgrim,* then he'll travel the world.'"

Pellegrino's parents are from the south of Italy, from the Naples area. And like many Italians of the fifties and sixties, they were unemployed, so they went abroad to look for work. They could have ended up anywhere but for better or for worse, they happened to move to the UK.

Pellegrino was born and raised in the UK in the city of Bath, which is ironically known as the Roman city of Bath. He grew up in a bicultural family where Italian culture and British culture were always at odds.

Now there's a pretty big difference between the Italians that emigrated to the States vs. the Italians that emigrated to Europe. The Italians who emigrated to the States did their very best to become Americans. They worked hard to embrace their Italian American identity, and they made it happen. Pellegrino says that America, being a *tabula rasa* sort of country where the "American Dream" exists, allowed for people to do what they wanted to do which made it easier for immigrant groups to assimilate.

On the other hand, Europe wasn't as forgiving to immigrants. According to Pellegrino, those who moved to Europe would forever remain foreigners. Europe was already steeped in centuries of history and traditions, which meant the host country would often already have a set way of doing things and stick to them. Meanwhile, the immigrants would hold on to their own traditions with the same vigor. As a result, there was hardly any chance of assimilating with the local people. Pellegrino suspects this is why the Italians who went to European countries like Germany and the UK did their very best to maintain their Italian culture, to the point of basically having as little to do with the local population as possible.

And so was the case with Pellegrino's father and mother. Pellegrino's parents, like many other Italians who emigrated to the UK, made sure that their kids stayed as close to their Italian culture as possible so that when they met other Italians, they could identify with them. The Riccardi household was basically a Little Italy. "I leave the door in the morning and I'm in England, then I come home through the same door in the evening and I'm in Italy," as Pellegrino described it. At home they spoke in

Italian, they ate Italian food, they grew up with Italian friends (who all came from the same village in Italy). Heck, when the Riccardis went to Italy on vacation, they would see all the same people, just in a hotter country. The only thing that was English in their house was the TV—his parents unfortunately couldn't do anything to change that. Though Pellegrino and his siblings grew up in England, it was as if they were raised in Italy. They were completely immersed in the Italian culture.

As great of a job Pellegrino's parents did with ensuring that the family stayed connected to their Italian roots, they began to grow more distant from the local British culture. Though they had lived in England for years, it was as if they were foreigners. This showed itself in their English skills... or rather, their *lack* of English skills. They spoke terrible English, and Pellegrino was basically their translator. His parents didn't mix with the local Brits due to the language and cultural barriers. But because they never exposed or immersed themselves in the local culture, they never got to learn how to overcome those barriers. It was a vicious cycle that prevented them from ever feeling integrated.

Throughout his childhood, Pellegrino worked hard to act as the bridge between his Italian parents and their British surroundings. Every day, he would accompany his father to important places like the bank, the insurance company, and the doctor's office. This was in the seventies and eighties, way before the internet. You couldn't just make transactions or purchases online—you had to stand in line and go see somebody in person and talk to them. Even to go to the shop and buy something like a sofa, Pellegrino had to be there to translate and relay his father's blunt and inadequate English in a way that was polite to the British shopkeepers. Pellegrino was a middleman between two starkly different cultures. He was his father's cultural broker.

This was quite common for children of immigrants—translating for their parents, filling out their financial paperwork, answering phone calls from agencies. "If you think about it, it can be quite a humiliating thing for the parents to go through," Pellegrino explained to me. "Their child is holding their hand, not the other way around. In cultures where the man is supposed to be the patriarch looking after his family and suddenly his kid is looking after him in the shop and translating 'sofa' and 'taxes' for him, it makes the man feel helpless to say the least. It's not easy for him." The honor of being the head of the family is torn away as a result, and Pellegrino realizes this particularly caused his father unending stress.

Pellegrino's father had a hard time navigating his way around this strange British culture that stood in stark contrast to his own Italian culture, and it only got harder when Pellegrino left Bath to pursue higher studies in Leeds. As Pellegrino's father grew older and his health began to deteriorate, trips to the doctor's office became routine. He developed hypertension, and his doctor prescribed him pills to take each morning.

But Pellegrino's father didn't feel like the medication was helping, so instead of taking one pill a day as prescribed, he would take two. When Pellegrino found out, he chided his father.

"Why are you doing that?"

"The one pill wasn't enough. I feel better taking two."

"But that's not the point. You've got to tell the doctor that you're changing the dose. Otherwise, it can kill you."

Pellegrino had a point. By taking two pills instead of one, the extra medication could cause his father's blood pressure to drop to a dangerously low level, and the doctor wouldn't know why.

"I didn't say anything because I didn't want to offend the doctor," said Pellegrino's father.

In Italian culture, the title "doctor" was a very revered title. As Pellegrino put it, doctors were equivalent to God and so their word was to be respected. In a culture where the doctor is so highly respected, it's almost impossible for patients to disagree with the doctor. It's very much a "you listen to me and accept what I say" kind of culture, which made sense given the years of schooling and education required to earn the title of "doctor."

In Anglo-Saxon cultures, the "doctor" title is still respected, but the stereotypical UK or US doctor is imagined as "burnt out and overworked, as someone who's really doing their best but is understaffed and underfunded," in Pellegrino's words. There's more freedom in these cultures to question the doctor and openly ask, "Are you sure about that?" and "Could I get a second opinion?" But in high-context hierarchical cultures that regard doctors with much respect and reverence, there isn't that freedom to question the doctor so openly.

So, the patients do it secretly...very secretly. Not wanting to offend the all-knowing doctor, they respond with the classic head nod and "okay." And then, they go home and verify the info for themselves and make changes as they see fit. This was exactly what Pellegrino's father did for years. He nodded "okay" to the doctor, went home, and took his own dosage as he saw fit. Thank goodness he finally told someone about it.

As soon as Pellegrino found out, he immediately called the doctor to inform him. "My father has been taking a different dose from what you prescribed because he feels it is not helping, but he didn't want to offend you by saying so."

It turned out that the doctor was anything but offended. In fact, it made his job much easier to know the new dose Pellegrino's father was taking and to understand why he was reluctant to say so. But because Pellegrino's father was so reluctant to expose himself to the local British culture, he could not communicate openly with his own doctor. He was unable to get beyond his cultural perception of "offending" the doctor. He needed his son to step in for him.

From this experience, Pellegrino realized the danger in failing to expose oneself to different cultures and adapt as needed. What is taken for granted in one culture could be unknown in another, preventing open communication as a result. Pellegrino went on to study Teaching English as a Second Language at the University of Oxford so he could help individuals like his father navigate the language and cultural barriers that come with being an immigrant in an English-speaking Anglo-Saxon country.

Some years later, Pellegrino met the love of his life, a beautiful Norwegian lady. He moved to Norway where he eventually settled down with his new family. Norway was unlike anything he had experienced as an Italian raised in the UK. Pellegrino was a playful and boisterous spirit that enjoyed friendly banter (thanks to his Italian upbringing), while Norwegians were a lot quieter and more reserved. When he moved to Norway, the first thing he did was learn the language, even though Norwegians speak English quite well. "I was determined to learn Norwegian and really understand them," he explained. "If I was not going to like them, at least I was doing it based on knowledge rather than prejudice."

Pellegrino, from the experiences of his parents and his childhood, learned the importance of exposing and adapting oneself to diverse cultures and viewpoints. With this mantra, he successfully runs his own consulting company, Pellegrino Consulting, that provides training to help people adapt in multicultural settings in order to collaborate more effectively. "The only way to communicate well and learn from each other is to *expose* yourself, to make yourself open and vulnerable to your surroundings," he tells his clients who seek his advice on cross-cultural communication. He aspires to create a global culture, one that takes the best parts of each culture and combines them into one.

Meanwhile, Pellegrino's father has since come a long way since his doctor fiasco. With the guidance of his kids, he has learned to communicate more openly and frankly with his doctor about his concerns. Sure, he still goes through some cultural mishaps, like the time he misunderstood his Norwegian daughter-in-law's invitation to go for a walk in the forest. A walk in the forest is a perfectly normal thing in Norway, where forests cover almost half the country. Accordingly, locals associate the Norwegian forest with fresh air, skiing, nature, elks, and other pleasant things. But for an Italian (particularly a Southern Italian) who comes from a culture that associates forests with rather gruesome events like kidnappings and whatnot, an invitation to walk in the forest naturally receives a response of fear and confusion. But despite these cross-cultural mishaps, Pellegrino's father is more willing to expose himself to the local culture and learn about the place where he lives, thanks to the encouragement of his son. He's putting in the effort where it matters most.

* * *

When Pellegrino first shared his father's story with me, I realized that I had experienced a similar version of this story many times before. Every year, my family has a fight about getting my dad to go to the doctor for his yearly checkup. It always happens at the end of the summer, after months of couch-potatoing and eating fried *bajjis* and *punugulu* and ice creams. "I feel fine" is the logic my dad often uses to try and escape from his appointments. "I'm taking your Amma's Vitamin D tablets for good measure," he offers as retribution. I usually then launch into a long lecture afterward about how he still has to get his blood pressure and cholesterol checked. I tell him it isn't a good idea to be taking pills that aren't prescribed for him specifically because they can have unwanted effects on the body's different systems, even if they're "just vitamins." He then proceeds to change the topic.

Though I had always known to some extent that my parents didn't like going to the doctor's, I realized I had never actually sat down with them and learned why. It wasn't until I started writing this book that I took the opportunity to talk with them about it and understand where they were coming from.

One blaring reason was the cost. To my parents, it seemed ridiculous to pay an eighty-dollar copay and seven-thousand-dollar yearly deductible for a mere ten minutes of the doctor telling them their blood pressure and cholesterol was normal. "I already knew I was healthy," my dad would probably say in response.

Another important reason, however, was their belief that the doctors wouldn't understand them. My parents would never tell their doctor about the various herbal medicines and supplements they took each day. They never bothered to because they figured the doctor either wouldn't understand what they were or would tell my parents to stop taking them. So, rather than discuss it with their doctor and have a conversation about it, they would just nod and then come home and take their own medicines and supplements as they saw fit. Just like Pellegrino's father, they didn't feel they had the liberty (or the time) to openly question the doctor and communicate their perspectives. In either case, it wasn't really the fault of the doctor or of our parents. It was, rather, a reasonable consequence of the cultural barriers and time restraints that had prevented our parents from being able to communicate openly with their doctor.

Pellegrino's story highlights an important, but often overlooked role of cultural brokers. We so often tend to think of cultural brokers as ones who educate the doctors and healthcare providers about the patient's cultural background and teach them how to adapt their care to fit the patient's beliefs. But just as cultural brokers work to help providers adapt to the patient's culture, they also work to help patients adapt to the culture of healthcare and the culture of the host country. Brokers help patients adapt their ways to fit the new culture they are now a part of. They help them find a healthy balance between living in these two cultures at once.

This describes the process of acculturation, or "the changes in beliefs, values, identity, or behaviors such as language, customs, diet, or social relationships that occur in minority-culture individuals (immigrant or indigenous) as a result of prolonged contact with the majority culture" (Boas, 1888). Sometimes, this process of acculturation is reflected in the way an individual speaks or dresses (i.e., their external behavior). Other times, it happens at a deeper psychological level and encourages change in an individual's thoughts and expectations.

The ethics behind acculturation is a tricky subject. Some argue that acculturation is a one-way ticket to losing one's identity entirely. Others believe that acculturation is a healthy and necessary process of adapting to one's surroundings to ensure that one's culture survives in an otherwise foreign environment. While I once strongly believed the former, reflecting upon the story of how Donya (our clinic's Mongolian interpreter) helped Enkhee with the Pap smear has led me to consider the real answer might be somewhere closer to the middle.

In fact, acculturation was at the root of how Donya helped Enkhee overcome her fear of the doctor. By encouraging Enkhee to open up about her cosmetic surgery, Donya helped Enkhee adapt her own preexisting impression of doctors to be more positive. She encouraged change in Enkhee's thoughts and expectations about the healthcare culture.

When Donya first moved to the Bay Area, she was working as a health worker at the local city hospital. Her job was largely centered around interviewing new immigrants, asylees, and refugees who came to the hospital for care. One particular patient interview she still remembers vividly was with a Mongolian mother (let's call her Alta) who came in with her young son.

When Donya walked into the patient room, she found Alta's son standing on the exam table. He jumped off with great force and landed in front of his mother.

"Hey, you shouldn't stand on the table," Donya intervened. "You'll hurt yourself!"

Donya then looked to Alta, who sat calmly in the patient chair and smiled proudly at her dear son. Her son was the tough boy in class, and his masculinity at such a young age was something that Alta (like many other Mongolian mothers) took pride in. Donya suspects this is a significant reason behind why domestic violence is so common in Mongolian families, with around one in three Mongolian women being victims of domestic violence (IDLO, 2020).

Donya began to interview Alta for her social and medical history, asking her questions like, "When did you move to the US?" and "What is your home life like?" As Alta shared her answers with Donya, the son walked up to his mother and began to pull on her hair. Alta didn't even move. She continued to answer Donya's questions as if nothing out of the ordinary was happening.

After Donya was finished with collecting Alta's history, the doctor came in to do the physical checkup. He took out his stethoscope and began to listen to Alta's lung sounds, when all of a sudden, they heard a shriek. The son began to run in circles in the middle of the room, yelling at the top of his lungs while the doctor was attempting to listen through his stethoscope. Donya had never seen such a rowdy kid before.

Donya looked at Alta, who finally intervened and said to her son, "Shhh quiet."

To Donya's and the doctor's absolute horror, the son screamed and straight up kicked his mother in the chin. The shocking part was that Alta wasn't even surprised. She just sat quietly, not saying a word.

Unable to stand the son's unacceptable behavior anymore, Donya stood up and intervened. She cornered the son and towered over him as she pointed her finger at him.

"I am the boss," Donya assertively told him. The son stopped screaming and looked up at Donya, eyes wide. "That means you do what I tell you to do. No screaming. No jumping. No kicking your mother. No crawling. You have to sit here *quietly*."

To everyone's surprise, the son listened and sat quietly on the exam table. Donya then turned to Alta and said, "Look around. Every single room here has a mother and child. Do you see anyone else running and screaming like your son is doing? No. That means your child is different."

The pride in Alta's smile faded as she realized how her son was the only child there that was behaving like this, and how he immediately listened when Donya said no.

As Donya was a mother herself, she knew the value of disciplining children from a young age. She understood the cultural barriers many Mongolian mothers faced in failing to discipline their sons. She instructed Alta, "When you discipline, you must say in a very calm voice: 'Hey honey, you're doing wrong.' And if they are trying to threaten you, get down to eye level with them and look straight into their eyes and say, 'I am the boss. You cannot win over me.' You do this one time, two times, and that's it. Now you're the boss."

Donya's role as a cultural broker was not just to make excuses for Alta's son's behavior by explaining to the doctor that this was a cultural pattern in Mongolian families. Her role was just as importantly focused on helping Alta adapt her parenting methods so her son would grow up to be a good member of society. There was value in recognizing what parts of a culture should be preserved versus what should be discarded, and Donya understood that the permissive parenting of Mongolian sons was one that had to go. By encouraging adaptation on the individual scale, with one patient at a time, Donya is able to create lasting positive cultural change without stripping the culture of its original roots.

CHAPTER 9

BALANCING ACT

"It is not easy to be stranded between two worlds. The sad truth is that we can never be completely comfortable in either world."

— SHARON KAY PENMAN

Dr. Neelima Chu comes from a family of physicians. Her mom (an OB-GYN) and dad (a venereologist) would spend long hours working at their clinic in Andhra Pradesh in the late seventies. Neelima's mom was a house surgeon, which meant she lived on the hospital's property and would be on call at all hours. Three-year-old Neelima would spend her playtime roaming around the hospital and making conversation with the physicians and patients. The residents and medical students were her family, and the hospital was her home. As Neelima shares, "Medicine was all I ever knew."

Some years later, her parents decided to move to the US for a change of pace. Neelima was ten years old at the time. Her mom and dad applied to and were accepted into their top choice residency programs (anesthesiology and psychiatry respectively) and began the long hard journey of completing their training while simultaneously raising two kids and running a household in an entirely new country. Neelima learned to cook at a very young age because she was the only one at home to make food when both of her parents were on call. And when Neelima's mom was chief resident in her final year, Neelima would often help her make the call schedule.

Naturally, Neelima was drawn to medicine from a young age and was motivated to pursue this profession when she fell in love with her physiology class in college. Neelima attended medical school at University of Vermont, where she met her now-husband and practicing pediatrician, Dr. Brian Chu.

Though Neelima was born in India and lived there for ten years, she has spent most of her life in America and considers herself to be just as American as she is Indian. Neelima now practices as an endocrinologist in San Diego, California. Because of the location of Neelima's practice, she tends to see a lot of young newly immigrated NRIs (non-resident Indians) that work at Qualcomm, a multinational software company that is headquartered in San Diego.

A lot of these NRIs tend to look for an Indian doctor, for someone who looks like them and will understand their unique struggles and way of life. So, when they find Neelima's profile and see she speaks Telugu, they are automatically drawn to choose her as their provider with the expectation that she will understand them and their situations more easily than a non-Indian provider.

Unfortunately, it isn't easy for Neelima when her patients walk in the door with such high expectations of her. She has to explain where "Chu" (her Vietnamese last name) comes from. She has to prove her fluency and expertise in Telugu. "I find it a little difficult, because now all of a sudden I'm expected to be more Indian than I am," Neelima shared with me. Being a part of two different cultural worlds and being held to such starkly different cultural expectations, no wonder she feels torn. And when she is unable to meet these expectations her patients hold either consciously or unconsciously, she worries about losing her patients' trust.

The expectations go both ways. Neelima admits she grows defensive when her patients begin throwing American healthcare under the bus by saying things like, "Well in India this doesn't happen" or "Why didn't you order this test for me? My doctor in India ordered it." Perhaps Neelima wouldn't have expected so much from other Americans, but she instinctively holds her fellow Indian co-ethnics to a different standard. Neelima holds her NRI patients to a more American standard while they hold her to a more Indian standard, neither being necessarily better than the other. "It's a double-edged sword," Neelima says. "I think they expect more from me and I expect more from them."

It seems as though these expectations arise from either side due to an *appearance* of shared culture, rather than a shared culture itself. "Our first receivers of information are our eyes. That's why we make judgment calls instantly when we see people," cross-cultural communications expert Pellegrino Riccardi explains. "When you see the same type of skin color, the same nose shape, the same eyes, and you identify with them on a physical basis, you certainly assume you'll identify with them on a deeper cultural and psychological level. That's not always the case, especially if they've grown up in another country."

Sure enough, Neelima and her patients both expect more from each other on the basis of shared appearance, for example, "You're brown and I'm brown therefore, you should understand where I'm coming from." But that is precisely where the danger lies. Neelima, though Indian by ethnicity, has not necessarily lived and experienced the exact same Indian culture her NRI patients have lived and experienced. She grew up almost entirely in the States, while her NRI patients immigrated here only a few years ago. Neelima is a doctor while her NRI patients are mostly all engineers. Neelima fell in love with and married her medical school classmate while many of her NRI patients had their marriages arranged by their parents. Despite coming from quite distinct cultures, Neelima and her patients each carry unrealistic expectations for each other solely based on their shared outer appearance.

When I asked Pellegrino if he had any insight into why this was the case, he explained to me: "It's not always a given that it's easy to communicate with people in the same culture because national culture is just one layer of many layers of culture. You will have more in common between a Singaporean surgeon and a Brazilian surgeon than a Brazilian surgeon and Brazilian football player. There are professional cultures, national cultures, regional cultures, and more. Culture is ultimately a group phenomenon, and it depends on how you define the group."

In fact, Pellegrino saw this phenomenon firsthand in his own immigrant family. "Our parents tried to keep us in touch with our Italian background so that when we met other Italians, we could identify with them," he shared with me. "But while I was able to identify with my Italian background, my sister wasn't. Oh, she was much more British than me. I was more attached to the home country and spoke the language better. I clicked with people when I went back to Italy, much more than my sister who was more British. My family was often disappointed with her."

Prithvi Mavuri, the Internal Medicine resident who took care of the Telugu patient with the GI bleed in Chapter Two, offered a unique perspective on this concept. "If you think about it, it's like when a white guy is marrying into an Indian family. On one hand you have the brown guy who is Indian by race, but knows nothing about his culture. On the other hand, you have the white guy who is so enamored by Indian culture and makes the effort to speak the language and learn the culture when coming into the family. Once the family gets past the outward impression of the guy being white, it becomes easier for them to digest because it's not just the race that matters. It's more about being culturally aware and sensitive."

This all goes to show an important point: culture is not genetic. Rather, culture is learned behavior that is passed down from generation to generation and changes over time. Yet, we so often associate culture and diversity with one's appearance rather than with this learned behavior that changes with time, place, and context. And this was precisely what led to these mutually unfulfilled expectations by both Neelima and her patients. There is more to culture than what meets the eye.

* * *

I decided to ask Chaitanya Patel, the Internal Medicine resident who helped the Hindi patient with anemia in

Chapter Three, if he had ever found it difficult to provide care for patients who share his culture. In response, he shared with me a recent story about an elderly Indian patient of his (let's call him Bharat) who was hospitalized with COVID. Bharat had been having difficulty with breathing on his own, and it got to the point where he was constantly short of breath and unable to fill his lungs completely. He was brought to the ICU and placed on CPAP (continuous positive airway pressure), a type of breathing support. With CPAP, the patient starts each breath themselves and the machine helps them complete the breath by filling their lungs with the needed oxygen. Bharat was lucky he didn't require an invasive form of ventilation, which would have required sedating him and sticking a large tube down his windpipe to push air from the ventilator into his lungs.

Bharat's family was worried about his prognosis, but they weren't allowed to come in to see him due to safety and exposure concerns. The doctors normally request only one person from each patient's family act as the point person to relay information to the rest of the family members. This is so the doctors have a clear and efficient mode of communication with the family about the patient's progress. But in Bharat's case, there were three to four different family members calling Chaitanya multiple times a day, wanting full updates on every single detail about Bharat's progress.

Chaitanya was worn thin from having to repeat the same explanation multiple times per day to these family members, but he also felt guilty about refusing to do so. On the phone, the family members called him *"beta"* (a term of endearment in Hindi often used by elder family members to call a younger person) and thanked him profusely for what he was doing.

Knowingly or unknowingly, Bharat's family members were taking advantage of their shared cultural connection with Chaitanya in order to win more of his time and attention. Chaitanya understood this wasn't inherently bad, and the family was doing this out of concern and worry for Bharat. It was a culturally acceptable thing to do. But at the same time, this had never happened with any other family. Other families followed the rules and appointed one point person as was instructed by the ICU doctors, but Bharat's family didn't seem to heed these rules.

It was Chaitanya's responsibility to treat Bharat's family in the same way he treated all the other patient families. He couldn't play favorites just because they shared a cultural connection. "It's overwhelming because there's other families that also needed to be talked to," Chaitanya shared with me. "I can't just be sitting there talking to the same five people in a family every single day for twenty minutes each." It just wasn't feasible or fair.

Unlike many other COVID patients who were brought to the ICU, Bharat was there for quite a long time, several weeks in fact. Chaitanya was so exhausted by the multitude of daily conversations happening with each of Bharat's family members, that it came to a point where he had to have a discussion with them. He spoke to Bharat's daughter over the phone one afternoon.

"I understand that your family is concerned, but we have limited time and resources to where we can only speak to one family member per day," Chaitanya explained. "If your family wants to get on a group call

all at once, I'd be happy to talk with you guys. But I can only designate one phone call at a time."

The daughter understood, and she thanked Chaitanya for all he did for them. They had reached a cordial resolution to the entire issue, yet Chaitanya couldn't help but reflect this was something he had never experienced with his other patients' families. It may or may not have been solely due to their shared cultural connection, but it certainly played a part.

Whether it is a provider caring for a same-culture patient, or a separate cultural broker acting as a middleman between patient and provider, boundaries must be drawn and enforced in order to ensure the fairest care and sustainable distribution of resources. Intentionally or unintentionally, Chaitanya was put into the role of cultural broker because his patient saw a shared culture with him. But Chaitanya felt responsible for this role because there was no one else to do it. As a result, he ended up taking on too much in his attempts to be accommodating for his patients. How fair was it to Chaitanya to have to fill this gap? Would his white colleagues have the same expectation from their patients, or did they have more of a choice to say no in instances of trying to bridge these cultural gaps?

Based on Chaitanya's experiences, as well as the experiences of many other physicians from different ethnic and cultural backgrounds, it seemed logical that these physicians would be experiencing more burnout than their white colleagues. After all, it is the physicians from minority ethnic groups that tend to experience more bias, cultural fatigue, conflicting expectations, and other factors that contribute to burnout.

I was surprised to find this was, in fact, *not* the case. According to a 2020 cross-sectional national study by Dr. Luis Garcia et. al., physicians from ethnic minority groups (incl. Hispanic, Black, and Asian) actually reported *lower* rates of occupational burnout compared to white physicians. The study utilized the Maslach Burnout Inventory as the primary metric of burnout, which offers statements such as: "I would choose to become a physician again" and "My work schedule leaves me enough time for my personal/family life" to gauge burnout level. Physicians who mark "strongly disagree" or "disagree" in response to these questions would receive a high score of emotional exhaustion and depersonalization on the burnout scale.

How was it possible that minority physicians were reporting *lower* burnout rates? If physicians from ethnic minorities are experiencing more factors that lead to burnout compared to white physicians, then why are they reporting less burnout? While the sample size used in Garcia's study was not large enough to make sense of all the different factors at play in the ethnicity-burnout association, a few other researchers in the field have offered some theories. One particularly interesting theory posed by Dr. Joel Cantor, the Founding Director of the Center for State Health at Rutgers University, is while minority physicians may be exposed to more burnout-causing factors in the workplace, they report more favorable accounts of work-life balance due to stronger family support and community-oriented practices within these cultures. This suggests the significant role of the physician's cultural background and practices in contributing to resiliency in the workplace.

Another theory is graduating medical students from minority groups are far more likely to go on to serve minority patient populations in the future, suggesting physicians from minority groups have a "greater intrinsic motivation to address the needs of patients with complex social and health challenges" (Cantor, 2020). Because of this longstanding motivation, they are more likely to answer "strongly agree" to questions like "I would choose to become a physician again" in the Maslach Burnout Inventory. It seems that although life as a physician poses several challenges for those from cultural minority groups, these physicians are more likely to view their role's challenges as an important part of their identity.

* * *

Sirisha Narayana, the Internal Medicine hospitalist who revived her patient by calling her "Aunty" in Chapter Three, has spent a great deal of time reflecting upon her multitude of different identities and how they have shaped her role as a physician. Sirisha has always aligned strongly with her Indian identity. Though she was born and raised in Pennsylvania, she fondly remembers her family's summer trips to India, the warm conversations with her grandparents and extended family, the Telugu movies they watched, the food they ate, and the experiences they shared.

Sirisha was one of the few South Asian kids in her school while in Pennsylvania. But once she moved to the Bay Area in her teens, she was surrounded by many other brown-skinned dark-haired kids, and she felt right at home. She never recalled going through the classic "identity crisis" so many children of immigrants experience, probably because she was just like all the other kids around her. She spoke Telugu at home while her best friends spoke Hindi. She spent her weekends taking Carnatic (South Indian classical music) vocal lessons while her classmates spent their Saturday mornings in Chinese school. She went to India during summer vacations to visit her family while her friend went to Israel to see his family. Though she and her friends belonged to different cultures, they were "similarly different in their own cultural upbringing." Sirisha found strength and pride in her Indian identity, and it grew to become an important part of her.

That is, until she became a doctor. "Very quickly, I started living and breathing this profession," she shared. "And it's not just the years of training or the hours we spend at work. It's the language we speak. It's how we think, how we feel." Her identity as a physician only continued to grow stronger and stronger as it began to infiltrate the other parts of her life, like her "strange ability to eat standing up anywhere, or her instant comfort when talking with other doctors." In fact, she began to notice her other identities (even her dearly-held Indian identity) becoming secondary to her identity as a physician.

On an episode of *The Nocturnists* podcast, Sirisha narrates her experience of taking care of an elderly Indian patient and shares how it has helped her find balance among her identities. The patient (let's call her Bhanu) was transported to UCSF General Hospital for more advanced care. Within hours of arrival, Bhanu went into shock. Her team of doctors had an incredibly difficult time figuring out what was going on as Bhanu's condition grew worse day by day. Sirisha was worried. Bhanu was far sicker than she should have been. Sirisha was worried they were missing something crucial, and it was right under their nose.

Bhanu's fifty-year-old son Ravi came every so often to visit his mother, but his presence was minimal. He would commute back-and-forth between his mother's bedside and that of another sick relative in the East Bay. Sirisha remembers being somewhat irritated by Ravi's absence during what was a particularly difficult time for Bhanu.

On Sirisha's last day of service, Bhanu coded in the ICU. Sirisha called Ravi that morning and begged him to come see his mother for the last time. When he came, he seemed unsurprised and passive. Perhaps it was because Bhanu had been sick for so long that he knew the inevitable would happen sooner or later.

After realizing Bhanu's options were incredibly limited, even with prolonged life, her doctors changed her code status to DNR ("do not resuscitate"). As Bhanu's heart rate and blood pressure dropped, the medical team slowly began to filter out of the room. Sirisha was the last to leave. She lingered outside Bhanu's room for a bit longer and watched Ravi as he sat by his mother. Ravi had been passive the whole time his mother was in the ICU, showing no emotion or reaction. Sirisha wanted to see if he would at least react now.

Ravi sat next to his mother and brushed her hair behind her ear. He held her hand in his, and then he said one word.

Amma.

Sirisha remembers feeling the wind rush out of her in that moment. *Amma* is the Telugu word for mother. *Amma* is the word Sirisha uses to call her own mother. Sirisha's eyes began to fill with tears as she began to imagine the face of her mother, then of every Indian woman she knew, in Bhanu's place. These women were all *Ammas,* just as Bhanu was an *Amma,* just as Sirisha's own mother was an *Amma.*

Sirisha admits she has a particularly difficult time taking care of Indian women because of what she refers to as the "*Amma* factor." These women, these *Ammas,* look at Sirisha, their doctor, as a young Indian woman not all that different from their own daughters. In turn, Sirisha can't help but look at her patients, these older Indian women, as *Ammas.*

"As physicians, we all have a type of patient persona that strikes a chord with us," Sirisha shares. For Sirisha, the *Amma* is one such persona that strikes a chord. When she sees her own *Amma* or even herself reflected upon the patients she cares for, there's the slightest bit more emotional investment. It's the same sort of emotion one experiences when caring for a relative or friend. While it's good to be invested to a certain extent, it is important to stay balanced and to not get lost in that attachment. "You can't let it drag you down emotionally," Sirisha emphasizes. "The first step is recognizing it and checking yourself to make sure that you're practicing objective medicine, but also knowing when it's okay to blur that line a little bit."

And yet, despite the emotional challenge the *Amma* factor presents, Sirisha would not give up seeing her Indian patients for anything. While it is challenging to be caring for patients who remind you of yourself, Sirisha understands this balancing act isn't necessarily a bad thing. When she sees an elderly Indian patient, she can't help but be reminded that she is more than her identity as a doctor. By seeing herself and her family reflected in the patients she takes care of, she is reminded that she is also a daughter, an Indian, a woman, a wife. She is reminded "[she] is not just a doctor, but a great many things more."

CHAPTER 10

CROSSING CIRCLES

"The action most worth watching is not at the center of things, but where edges meet."

— ANNE FADIMAN, *THE SPIRIT CATCHES YOU AND YOU FALL DOWN*

Latha Panchap was a stellar medical student. She aced her USMLE Step 1 exams and breezed through her MS1 and MS2 years. Now, she was beginning her third year of medical school, which meant her first clinical clerkships... and her first pimping. Pimping, as those in the medical field fondly call it, is the process in which the senior-most physician (usually the attending physician) rather aggressively grills the students and junior residents on their medical knowledge, asking them various questions about the patient case in front of them during clinical rounds. The ones who answer the questions quickly and correctly earn the respect of the senior doctors, while those who do not fall behind in the ranks.

Latha knew all the answers, but she rarely spoke up. She figured her goal wasn't to show off her memory of the textbook. To Latha, what was more important was demonstrating her dedication to medicine through the time she spent with her patients and the thoroughness of her presentations to her attendings. Unfortunately, her attendings thought otherwise. As Latha shared on an episode of *The Nocturnists* podcast, one attending physician called her into his office one afternoon. "You seem to lack a basic level of confidence," he told her bluntly in his Eastern European accent. "I suggest you pursue a different career path entirely. Your personality won't serve you here." Latha cried to herself that night. By being quiet and reserved, she was assumed to be lacking in confidence, even though that wasn't the case.

If she wanted to excel in her clerkship years and receive solid recommendations from her superiors, she needed to do something differently. Latha resolved to change. She forced herself to participate intensely during the pimping sessions, making sure the attending knew she was not afraid to speak up. She was the first to arrive at the hospital and the last one to leave. She stayed late to personally sign out patients. She pressed her superiors for feedback on her performance. She went out of her way to print out the sheets for her attending, even going so far as to fold them exactly how he liked it.

She was more exhausted than she had ever been, but her newfound change did the trick and her evaluations skyrocketed. Her confidence and competency were through the roof. Still, it felt as though something was missing. Her fellow classmate sat down next to her one day during a break and said dejectedly, "I feel like these days, I don't volunteer to do anything for a patient unless I know that a resident or attending is watching me." Those words hit Latha like a brick.

Some days later, a new patient was brought onto their floor. Mr. Q was a fifty-nine-year-old man who had previously received radiation therapy for a cancer diagnosis and was now suffering from osteonecrosis of the jaw as a result. His jawbone was exposed, and he could barely move his mouth. His sentences came out as garbled noises. He was supposed to go to ENT for surgery, but he stayed on Latha's floor for pre-surgical imaging and stabilization. Mr. Q was 70 percent deaf, and he spoke a rare dialect of Cantonese called Toisan. It was difficult to find an interpreter that could speak Toisan and communicate between Mr. Q and his doctors. Even when they did manage to find an interpreter to help, it was hard to communicate given Mr. Q's difficulty hearing and his slurred speech.

Mr. Q stayed on their service for three weeks because his surgery kept getting delayed. Here was Mr. Q, stuck in a foreign country, lying in a strange-looking hospital bed, surrounded by voices speaking a language he didn't know. He had debilitating jaw and head pain every time he moved, and he couldn't tell anyone about it because no one could understand him. He spent his days looking gloomily out the window in his patient room.

Latha saw him every day, but she was caught in the daily whirlwind of pimping from her attendings and presentations to prepare and other patients to see. If she wanted to keep up the stellar recommendations from her attendings, she couldn't afford to spend more than a few minutes per day with Mr. Q. She often went to bed at night wondering whether he was still looking gloomily out of his window in that moment.

Latha saw him again the next day, only this time she gave his hand a small squeeze before she left his room.

He didn't move and continued to look gloomily out the window. Latha was torn. There was a small part of her had hoped he would reciprocate, but alas.

Latha no longer wanted to be the smartest and loudest student who constantly craved approval. She slowly stopped tagging along behind her attendings and folding their papers for them. Instead, she began to spend more and more time in Mr. Q's room, eventually checking in with him up to four times a day to give him company.

Beyond a thumbs up or thumbs down for his pain level, they could barely communicate with each other. Latha decided to print out a sheet of basic words in Cantonese characters with their English translations next to them, along with a diagram of the human body. He pointed to the word for pain, and then pointed to the body part where he was feeling the pain. He then gave a thumbs up or thumbs down to indicate how bad his pain was. Over time, their vocabulary grew. They incorporated new words and gestures for things like nausea, coughing, sleep, etc. that helped Latha learn more about his condition. It was through this unique language they created together that Latha was able to learn he had fallen on his way to the bathroom one night. He struggled on the floor for two minutes before forcing himself to get up and go back to bed. He didn't alert the nurses because he didn't realize he should, nor did he know how.

As Latha spent more days with him, Mr. Q spent less time looking out the window. He showed her pictures of himself before his cancer diagnosis, of his family in his home country, of his favorite foods and places. He started smiling. The day he went out to ENT for his surgery,

Latha squeezed his hand to say goodbye. And this time, he squeezed it back.

After his surgery, he was placed in subacute care, where his family was waiting for him. As Latha was saying goodbye to him, he handed her the papers they had used as their dictionary. He took her hands and touched them to his eyes as if to say, "Thank you."

Those few weeks were a rollercoaster for Latha. She was naturally a pretty quiet person who preferred not to be in the spotlight. She was told these were the qualities that would prevent her from succeeding in medicine, but her time with Mr. Q suggested otherwise. As important as it was that she was a confident and competent physician, it was the quiet and unassuming Latha that was the one to break down barriers and build connections with vulnerable patients like Mr. Q.

As heartwarming as her story was, I couldn't help but lament how Latha was forced to choose between being a competent medical student and being an advocate for her patients. Be it the limited hours she had with Mr. Q or the intensely high expectations of her attendings she had to meet, she faced multiple barriers that prevented her from fulfilling all the duties required by her. Perhaps if she also spoke Toisan or was familiar with Mr. Q's cultural background, she might have had an easier time being able to perform the many duties that were placed upon her. She had spent so much time working to understand Mr. Q's language and culture, working so hard to serve as his advocate, that she grew torn from her other duties as a clinician.

This is a dilemma providers have struggled with for years. According to a 2018 study by researcher Frederic

Michas, about one in every four primary care doctors spend less than twelve minutes with a patient. No wonder doctors are constantly straddling this fine line between establishing rapport with their patients and providing competent and efficient care. Though the two are very much tied together, the time and energy constraints of physicians never allow them to fulfill both comprehensively.

This is why cultural brokership is so important. The broker's entire job is to establish rapport between patients and doctors so doctors can focus more of their attention on providing necessary care. Perhaps the Toisan interpreter should have played a larger role in Mr. Q's care in order to facilitate communication across language and cultural barriers. Yet, despite not knowing the language or the culture, Latha was able to move past those barriers and establish a real connection with Mr. Q. She didn't need the interpreter in order to advocate meaningfully for Mr. Q. All she needed was for her attendings to give her the space to serve as a broker without penalizing her in other areas. Latha's story dug at the root of a question that lies at the center of this entire book: How much does it matter that the provider shares the same culture as their patient?

* * *

In May 2021, a fifty-six-year-old Muslim woman called Beevathu was admitted into the COVID-19 ward at Sevana Hospital in the Palakkad district of Kerala, India. Beevathu, who was critically ill from COVID-19 related pneumonia, was placed on a ventilator for over two weeks.

This type of invasive life-support, where a large tube is inserted through the patient's mouth into the windpipe, is often used as a last resort to help the patient breathe when they are unable to on their own. When on a ventilator, the patient cannot eat, drink, speak, or move. Sometimes, they are even sedated to prevent movement that might dislodge the tube from the windpipe.

None of Beevathu's family or friends were allowed inside to see her due to COVID-19 precautions. As a result, her doctors were the ones to take on the role of comfort and support her family would have otherwise provided. For over two weeks as Beevathu underwent treatment and ventilation, her son and son-in-law would come to the hospital, ignoring heavy rains and lockdown restrictions, in order to check on their mother. Even though they weren't allowed inside the hospital, they waited for hours in the parking lot just to see the doctor and inquire about Beevathu. They knew her condition wasn't going to improve, yet they came daily to meet the doctor and get some peace of mind that she was in the right hands.

Beevathu's condition continued to deteriorate despite her ventilation support. By May 17, her organs began to shut down. The doctors were afraid there was not much left they could do for her at this point. After discussing with Beevathu's family, they made the difficult decision to take her off the ventilator.

Her doctors stood around her helplessly as Beevathu gasped for air. One of her doctors, Dr. Rekha Krishnan, sensed she was struggling during her last moments, unable to leave peacefully. Though Hindu by faith, Dr. Krishnan leaned forward and softly recited the Islamic *Kalima Shahida* prayer into the patient's ear. This prayer is traditionally recited by Muslims at the time of one's death in order to ensure a peaceful transition from life.

What touched Dr. Krishnan most was that as she uttered the last words of the *shahida*, "*La ilaha illallah Muhammadur rasulullah*," Beevathu took her last breath and flatlined. "The way this happened made me feel that someone made me do it, like a divine intervention," Dr. Krishnan shared. "If her daughter or a family member was there, they too would have done the same thing. It was not a religious act, but a humanitarian one."

The episode had a profound impact on Dr. Krishnan, yet she chose to share it with no one but a colleague of hers, Dr. Mustafa. Dr. Mustafa was moved by Dr. Krishnan's incredible act of compassion and decided to share the story with his family and friends via a Facebook post. Little did either of them know that Dr. Mustafa's post about her would blow up overnight and become viral. Within hours, words of praise and appreciation began pouring in from around the world for Dr. Krishnan's exemplar gesture of humanity.

Dr. Krishnan, though born in Kerala, was raised in Dubai all her life. She grew up in and around cultural diversity as she fasted both for *Mandalam* (a forty-one day period of prayer and pilgrimage in Hinduism) and *Ramadan* (a month of worship and remembrance in Islam). She knew the customs and practices followed by Hindus and Muslims alike. "I was never discriminated against because of my faith when I was in the Gulf and I returned the respect when I got a chance," Dr. Krishnan told the *Times Now News*. "Chanting the *kalima* was a normal thing I would have done any other day if needed, just like a family member."

Dr. Krishnan's story was especially inspiring because of how rare it was. How often do you find a provider who is not just willing, but comfortable with performing the last rites of another culture and religion? It just so happened to work out in this case such that Dr. Krishnan was knowledgeable, comfortable, and welcome to chant the *kalima* for her patient. But what if the doctor *wasn't* comfortable performing the rites of a culture they didn't belong to, because it was against their own beliefs? Or what if the patient's culture was a closed one, such that those who didn't belong to that culture were not welcome to practice it? In such instances, who is the right person to be deemed a cultural broker?

Dr. Karen Sun, Chief of the Department of Pediatric Hospital Medicine at UCSF, believes the right candidates for cultural brokership fill a sort of gray area or middle ground between the patient's culture and the broader healthcare culture. It's close to impossible that a cultural broker shares the exact same culture as both the patient and the provider, hence why many brokers occupy this middle ground.

Culture exists in many concentric circles, so it is always challenging to be a perfect match in all senses of culture. For example, Mr. Singh (the Punjabi Sikh patient at the clinic where I work) and I both share a common Indian culture (occupying one large concentric circle). However, he embodies Sikh culture while I embody Hindu culture, and he speaks Punjabi while I speak Telugu (each occupying smaller distinct concentric circles). As such, finding where our circles cross while simultaneously recognizing our differences in our distinct concentric circles is important. "The best cultural brokers are people who have the knowledge and understanding of both sides," Dr. Sun explained to me. "These are often people that are respected within the community and also have the skills to navigate the complexities of healthcare."

Given all the requirements and responsibilities required to serve as a cultural broker, how do we go about implementing this position? Importantly, how feasible is it to appoint and designate a cultural broker to facilitate these patient interactions?

Many believe the time has come for official cultural brokers to be put into place in hospital systems in order to more evenly divide these responsibilities. In fact, this is something the UCSF hospital system has seen with their patients who come from other countries. "A lot of patients from Saudi Arabia with congenital heart disease are brought to UCSF for treatment," Dr. Sun shared with me. "They would hire somebody who is there full-time to act as a cultural ambassador, as someone who would liaison with these families and help them navigate our healthcare system." While this system worked very well, it was a costly operation that was only feasible for wealthy patient populations.

Others, noting these extreme costs involved with hiring official cultural brokers, instead suggest providers and hospitals partner with local cultural groups in the community to serve as freelance brokers, akin to how we have worked to battle the COVID-19 pandemic with the help of cultural leaders within our communities. Regardless of what the best solution might be, one thing is clear: we can't keep pushing providers like Latha and Chaitanya and Neelima into these roles. The role of cultural broker is too great to be placed upon any one person, especially one that is consumed with the many responsibilities that come with being a provider directly accountable for a patient's life. The only way to sustain cultural brokership is to make it a collaborative effort. By expanding cross-cultural training, exposing ourselves to different cultural backgrounds, and emphasizing cultural humility, we can all do our part to support our patients in culturally concordant ways.

* * *

The story of Reverend Gloria White-Hammond is one such story that exemplifies such cultural brokership. Gloria, lovingly known to her church community as "Pastor Gloria," has devoted much of her life to understanding the intersections of healing, spirituality, and end-of-life care. Pastor Gloria practiced as a pediatrician for over twenty-seven years and is now the co-pastor of Bethel AME Church in Boston, Massachusetts, as well as a resident practitioner in ministry studies at Harvard Divinity School. I first learned of Pastor Gloria as I was walking to work one morning listening to her feature on Duke Divinity School's podcast. As she discussed topics of African American spirituality and illness, Pastor Gloria shared one particularly memorable story about her experiences with cultural brokership.

In 2018, Gloria's friend (let's call her Margaret) was diagnosed with breast cancer. Margaret was scheduled to go to her first doctor's appointment after her diagnosis, and she was nervous to go on her own. Margaret asked Gloria if she would accompany her to the appointment. Gloria was not only a physician who was familiar with the proceedings of such a doctor's appointment, but as a longtime friend of Margaret, she was also familiar with Margaret's worries and concerns. Her knowledge of both the medical culture and Margaret's background would make her the perfect cultural broker.

As they sat in the waiting room, Gloria noticed how anxious Margaret looked.

"How are you feeling?" Gloria asked.

"Nervous."

Margaret, like Gloria, was a Black woman from the South (North Carolina to be exact), where religion and spirituality were a big part of the local lifestyle and culture. The most important thing for Margaret was to be sure that her doctor knew she loved Jesus and that God intended to heal her. Of the many wonderful qualities Gloria appreciated about her friend, the thing that really stood out to her was Margaret's unabashed boldness in declaring that Jesus was her Lord and Savior.

Gloria nodded. While such faith in God was typical in North Carolina where they were from, it was certainly quite unusual in Boston where they currently were. The receptionist called Margaret and Gloria to wait in the examining room for the nurse. As they waited, Margaret grew more and more nervous.

"Is it okay if we pray together, at least until the nurse gets here?" Margaret asked.

"Of course."

Margaret and Gloria prayed together. They prayed that the providers would understand her concerns, that her questions would be answered, and that God would guide her through this uncertain journey. At that point, the nurse entered the room and introduced herself to both

Margaret and Gloria. She had quite a stern expression on her face, like that of a principal who tolerates no nonsense from her students. She sat at the desk in front of the computer and positioned her hand over the keyboard to take note of Margaret's important history and physical information. The nurse went down the standard list of questions, and Margaret answered each one. Finally, the nurse arrived at this question on the list:

"What brings you to the doctor today?"

The simple answer would have been for Margaret to say, "breast cancer." But instead, Margaret launched into a testimony like it was, as Gloria put it, "a Friday night at Bethel Church."

"I was saved, sanctified, and filled with the Holy Ghost on April 23, 1989," Margaret answered. "I had been running with the devil, but after Jesus came into my life, I was running for Jesus. I know that God will heal me."

With that, Margaret threw her head back in the name of Jesus and shouted, "Hallelujah!"

Gloria, though a pastor at Bethel Church and quite spiritual herself, was nonetheless impressed by Margaret's answer. This wasn't North Carolina. This was Boston, and Bostonians just didn't do this sort of thing as far as Gloria knew. Gloria wondered how the nurse would react. Would she snicker? Would she roll her eyes and scoff? Or would she just pretend like Margaret didn't say anything?

To Gloria's surprise, none of those things happened. Something else happened instead. The nurse, who until then had been carrying a stern expression on her face, leaned over the desk towards Margaret and smiled.

"So, you're spiritual, right?" the nurse asked gently.

With that, the tightness that Margaret experienced, now and every time she had waited to see a doctor, was released. The wrinkles on her face faded away as the anxiety of the appointment left her. Margaret nodded, and a small smile appeared on her face. It was as though the thing that mattered most was heard and acknowledged at last.

What that nurse did was very simple, yet it was something that changed Margaret's entire experience and perspective surrounding healthcare. The nurse didn't share Margaret's spirituality and religion, but she didn't have to. A good cultural broker doesn't have to share the exact culture as the patient they work with. In fact, sharing the exact same culture can sometimes even be undesirable because the broker is then no longer in a position to act as a bridge between two different cultures, be it the patient vs. doctor culture, eastern vs. western culture, or spiritual vs. secular culture. The important point is that a good cultural broker is one who is willing to learn and understand how each culture operates and what challenges might be presented when both come into contact. The nurse *listened* to Margaret, and she strived to understand and acknowledge her fears and concerns. It is this humility and willingness to learn that can transform someone who knows nothing about a certain culture into the best cultural broker.

ACKNOWLEDGMENTS

A Case of Culture is, in many ways, the fruit of several serendipitous accidents. Though I have always loved storytelling, I never thought I could or would write a book. But somehow the stars aligned just right, and so began my journey to becoming an author. For this reason, I must first thank Lord Krishna for blessing me with the strength and opportunities to pursue this endeavor.

To my family, thank you for being there by my side at every step of this journey. I'm honestly surprised you didn't get sick of me FaceTiming you each day with endless book updates. Amma, I would never have found my love for storytelling if it weren't for the epic stories and *kathalu* you shared with us in our childhood. This book is in large part the fruit of your undying passion for our culture, language, and heritage. I hope I did it justice. Daddy, you have always taught me to work hard for work's sake and not for the fruits of my work. Your words have helped me get through some of the toughest parts of this journey, and I have no doubt they will continue to guide me in my future endeavors. Sujan, you are the bestest brother and friend anyone could ever ask for. I could always count on you to cheer me up and make me laugh when I was at my lowest. Ammamma and Tatayya, you have instilled within me a deep appreciation for our culture and our traditional ways. Thank you for letting me share your story with the world. I hope it will inspire others as much as it inspired me.

Thank you to my incredible interviewees, Hasan Gokal, Pellegrino Riccardi, Rob and Melodie Adams, Donya Tserendolgor, Priya Jaisinghani, Chinmaya Sharma, Prithvi Mavuri, Sirisha Narayana, Neelima and Brian Chu, Jacqueline Melecio, Sulagna Roy, Ryoko Chernomaz, Titi Mabogunje, Rao Kolusu, Karen Sun, Pamela Tipler, Janu Kanneganti, Shvetali Thatte, Raga Ramachandran, and all of the people whose stories and insights I share in my book. Your strength and vulnerability is unparalleled, and I know that so many of us have and will continue to be inspired by your stories.

A special thank you to Eric Koester, who first told me that if I put my whole heart into it, I really could write a book. Thank you for believing in me. To my editors, Paloma Wrisley and Katherine Mazoyer, thank you for helping bring my book's vision to life. Your patience, guidance, and wisdom has been instrumental in transforming my confused scribbles into a book worth reading. I'd also like to thank Brian Bies, John Saunders, Lisa Patterson, Amanda Brown, Gjorgji Pejkovski, Kierston Stephens, and the incredible team I've gotten to work with at the Creator Institute and New Degree Press. You've given me memories to last a lifetime.

A huge shoutout to Sumner Leyson and Micia Bonta, my fabulous Beta Readers. Thank you for your valuable feedback and endless encouragement throughout the revisions process. You helped reaffirm exactly how important it is that this book's message be shared with the world.

I have had many wonderful teachers and professors over the years who have meaningfully impacted my educational journey and taught me life lessons that I will carry with me forever. However, I must give my special thanks to one teacher in particular: my high school English teacher, Mr. Chris Harrington. Thank you, Mr. H, for helping me realize my potential as a thinker and writer.

To my extraordinary work-family at the San Francisco Free Clinic, without your guidance and mentorship, and without the special clinical experiences and patient interactions that SFFC has blessed me with, the inspiration behind this book would not exist.

To my fellow authors, Shysel Granados, Maham Kazmi, Samuel Dillow, Deepu Asok, Satish Shenoy, Jinny Uppal, and Patrick Lin, your companionship has been unlike any other. I am so grateful to have shared this rollercoaster ride with you. And a huge thank you to my fellow authors Shobha Dasari and Navya Janga, who were the first to inform me about this incredible opportunity to write this book with the Creator Institute.

To my amazing friends, thank you for your unconditional love, laughter, and shenanigans. Endless gratitude to my Parker gang, Mancave, Something Extra, the Federalist Party, d218, and Smart People. I'm so grateful that our friendship has remained just as strong despite time and distance. Thank you to my DJ squad for making the kickass mixes that kept me going during those early mornings of writing. And a huge thank you to my Clubhouse friends (shoutout to Telugu Tribe) for listening to my narrations of this book's early stories and offering much-needed humor and moral support.

Finally, I want to give a BIG thank you to this special group of individuals who pre-ordered a copy of my book and donated to my pre-launch campaign. Thank you for believing in me and my writing. This group includes: Robert & Melodie Adams, Harsh Agarwal, Eash Aggarwal, Joshua Altman, Udaya Amancharla, Lavanya Ande, Camille Arboles, Pilar Asensio, Eugene Auh, Scott Austin, Manaswini Avvari, Poshitha Bandarupalli, Vamsi Bhadriraju, Neha Bhatt, Nagesh Bidhurakanthu, Nerissa Bilar, Michelle Bonta, Matthew Campbell, Sarah Carter, Brian Cashin, Mallikarjunarao & Rajeswari Chalavadi, Ravinder Challa, Ryoko Chernomaz, Neelima & Brian Chu, Mary Chukwu, Madison Cupp-Enyard, Samuel Dillow, Ravi Divvela, Bill Draper, Jill Ann Duehr, Vishnu Duvuuru, David A Evans, Tomeka Frieson, Murali G, Visweswara Ganapathineedi, Patrick R Gaughen, Patricia and Richard Gibbs, Joe Gitchell, Hasan Gokal, Swarajyalakshmi Gollapudi, Raghava Gollapudi, Shysel Granados, Dan Grimm, Esin Gumustekin, Venu & Manjula Gunda, Medha & Vignesh Gunda, Ravi Hande, Canaan Harris, Anthony Hejduk, Hrishikesh, Patricia Hume, Manjeet K Hunjan, Kyle Hutzler, Dinesh Inavolu, Jevin James, Lionel Jin, Raghav Joshi, Ishita Juluru, Nirupam Kanagala, Lokesh Kanagala, Giri Karyamapudi, Sidd Kasi, Srijay Kasturi, Maham Kazmi, Seema Khurana, Sri Kodali, Eric Koester, Udaya Sai Kumar Kollipara, Navya Koppusetty, Prem Kumar, Glover Lawrence, Abbey Levantini, Sumner Leyson, David G Litt, Stephanie Malta, Ravi Meda, Mohith Medasani, Jahnavi Meka, Krishna Mendu, Ferozuddin Mojadedi, Srihari Mupparaju, Krishna Musunuru,

Nageswararao & Lokesh Nagineni, Sridhar Namburi, Krishnarao & Madhavi Nandipati, Srinivasa & Sunitha Nandipati, Sujan Venkata Nandipati, Jorge Nunez, Sarah & Amy Ogle, Vijay Parthasarathy, Maryam Chloe Pervaiz, Sricharan Pusala, Fatima Qazi, Sriram Ranga, Raj Rao, Subbarao Ravuri, Meghana Reddy, Nicholas Rogozinski, Edwin Rosete, Ali Rupani, Harinandan Sainath, Anil Sankaramanchi, Kameswara Rao Saripella, Joseph Severini, Swapna Sharma, Sheila, Satish Shenoy, Suraj Srinivasan, Krishnamurthy Srinivasan, Tej Sutariya, Uma Talagadadivi, Praveen Tammana, Belinda Tan, Andreas Towers, Jinny Uppal, Gopikrishna Vadlamudi, Saikrishna Reddy Vanukuri, Satish Vattikuti, Venkat Vempati, Venu Vittaladevuni, Weitai, Dwight Kim & Donna Padgett Wimpey, Joseph Wood, Joanna Wu, Vikas Yadlapalli, Subbarao & Sunitha Yakkala, Sri Yalamanchi, Stacey Zoyiopoulos, and David Zuckerman.

To all of you who have made *A Case of Culture* possible, I want to thank you from the bottom of my heart. This is for you.

APPENDIX

INTRODUCTION

- Ekor, Martins. "The growing use of herbal medicines: issues relating to adverse reactions and challenges in monitoring safety." *Frontiers in Pharmacology 4*, no. 177 (2014): https://doi.org/10.3389/fphar.2013.00177.

- Jezewski, M. A. "Culture Brokering in Migrant Farm Worker Health Care." *Western Journal of Nursing Research* 12, no. 4 (1990): 497–513.

- Linzer, M., A. Bitton, S.P. Tu, M. Plews-Ogan, K.R. Horowitz, M.D. Schwartz, et. al. "The End of the 15-20 Minute Primary Care Visit." *Journal of General Internal Medicine* 30, no. 11 (2015): 1584–1586. https://doi.org/10.1007/s11606-015-3341-3.

- U.S. Census Bureau. 2000. *United States Census 2000. Profile of General Demographic Characteristics*. Washington, D.C.: U.S. Census Bureau.

CHAPTER 1: THE WELL FROG

- Baisch, Mary J., Pang C Vang, Beth R. Peterman. "An Exploration of Hmong Women's Perspectives on Cancer." *Asian Nursing Research* 2, no. 2 (2008): 82-91. doi: 10.1016/S1976-1317(08)60032-8.

- Colby, Sandra L. & Jennifer M. Ortman. *Projections of the Size and Composition of the U.S. Population: 2014 to 2060.* Washington DC: US Census Bureau, 2015.

- Csordas, Thomas J. "The Sore That Does Not Heal: Cause and Concept in the Navajo Experience of Cancer." *Journal of Anthropological Research* 45, no. 4 (1989): 457-485. http://www.jstor.org/stable/3630519.

- Darsha, Adrija K. & Philip R. Cohen. "New Onset of Linear Purpura on the Back: Coining Therapy-Associated Ecchymoses." *Cureus* 12, no. 6 (2020): doi:10.7759/cureus.8833.

- Davies, Wade. "Healing Ways: Navajo Health Care in the Twentieth Century." *Journal of American History* 89, no. 2 (2002): 680-681. https://doi.org/10.2307/3092270.

- Morse A. 2003. *Language Access: Helping Non-English Speakers Navigate Health and Human Services.* National Conference of State Legislature's Children's Policy Initiative.

- NCCC (National Center for Cultural Competence). *Bridging the Cultural Divide in Health Care Settings: The Essential Role of Cultural Broker Programs.* Washington DC: Georgetown University Center, 2004.

- Nielsen-Bohlman, L., AM Panzer, DA Kindig. *Health Literacy: A Prescription to End Confusion.* Washington (DC): National Academies Press, 2004.

- Strom, Karen. "Navajo Ceremonials." Accessed May 6, 2021. http://www.hanksville.org/voyage/navajo/ceremonials.php3.

- Tan, AK. & P. Mallika. "Coining: An Ancient Treatment Widely Practiced Among Asians." *Malaysian Family Physician: The Official Journal of the Academy of Family Physicians of Malaysia* 6, no. 2-3 (2011): 97–98.

- Vivekananda. "Sisters and Brothers of America." (speech), Sept. 11, 1893. Parliament of World's Religions, Chicago. Transcript, Complete Works of Swami Vivekananda.

CHAPTER 2: A SHORE OF FAMILIARITY

- Anderson, Steven, Morgan Gianola, Jenna M Perry, and Elizabeth A Reynolds Losin. "Clinician–Patient Racial/Ethnic Concordance Influences Racial/Ethnic Minority Pain: Evidence from Simulated Clinical Interactions." *Pain Medicine,* 21, no. 11 (2020): 3109–3125. https://doi.org/10.1093/pm/pnaa258.

- Singh, Rupinder. "11 Things You Wanted to Know About My Turban But Were Too Afraid to Ask." *The Mashup Americans* (blog). 2021. http://www.mashupamericans.com/issues/is-it-hot-under-there/.

- Wensley, Cynthia, Ann McKillop, Mari Botti, and Alan F. Merry. "Maximising Comfort: How do Patients Describe the Care That Matters? A Two-Stage Qualitative Descriptive Study to Develop a Quality Improvement Framework for Comfort-Related Care in Inpatient Settings." *BMJ Open* 10, no. 5 (2020): https://doi.org/10.1136/bmjopen-2019-033336.

CHAPTER 3: THE CHAMELEON EFFECT

- Hofstede Insights. "Country Comparison." Accessed Oct. 10, 2021. https://www.hofstede-insights.com/.

- Jalil, Majid and Rosslynne Freeman. "Research: Culture in Medicine and Healthcare." Accessed Feb. 3, 2021. https://www.cultureandmedicine.org/research.

- Jalil, Majid, Rosslynne Freeman, and Stephen Brigley "Support Refugee Doctors." *Education for Primary Care* 18, no. 6 (2007): 759-762. doi: 10.1080/14739879.2007.11493615.

- Joseph, Sinu. *Rtu Vidya: Ancient Science Behind Menstrual Practices.* Chennai: Notion Press, 2020.

- Narayana, Sirisha. "A Great Many Things More." Feb. 6, 2018. In *The Nocturnists.* Produced by Emily Silverman. Podcast, MP3 Audio. https://thenocturnists.com/season1/2018/5/8/2-a-great-many-things-more.

CHAPTER 4: KEEPING SECRETS AND BREAKING TRUST

- Brandt, Allan M. "Racism and Research: The Case of the Tuskegee Syphilis Study." *The Hastings Center Report* 8, no. 6 (December 1978): 21–29. doi:10.2307/3561468.

- Brandt, Allan M. *No Magic Bullet: A Social History of Venereal Disease in the United States since 1880.* New York: Oxford University Press; 1987.

- Brown, DeNeen L. "'You've Got Bad Blood': The Horror of the Tuskegee Syphilis Experiment." *Washington Post,* May 16, 2017. https://www.washingtonpost.com/news/retropolis/wp/2017/05/16/youve-got-bad-blood-the-horror-of-the-tuskegee-syphilis-experiment/.

- CDC (Centers for Disease Control and Prevention). "The U.S. Public Health Service Syphilis Study at Tuskegee." Accessed April 21, 2021. https://www.cdc.gov/tuskegee/timeline.htm.

- Duff-Brown, Beth. "The shameful legacy of Tuskegee syphilis study still impacts African-American men today." *Stanford Health Policy.* January 6, 2017. https://healthpolicy.fsi.stanford.edu/news/researchers-and-students-run-pilot-project-oakland-test-whether-tuskegee-syphilis-trial-last.

- Ebright, John R., Togoo Altantsetseg, Ravdan Oyungerel. "Emerging Infectious Diseases in Mongolia." *Emerging Infectious Diseases* 9, no. 12 (2003): 1509-1515. doi:10.3201/eid0912.020520.

- Garcia, Thea. "What is the HIPAA Privacy Rule?" *Reciprocity,* November 11, 2019. https://reciprocity.com/resources/what-is-the-hipaa-privacy-rule/.

- Hamel, Liz, Ashley Kirzinger, Cailey Muñana, Mollyann Brodie. "KFF COVID-19 Vaccine Monitor: December 2020." *Kaiser Family Foundation (KFF),* December 15, 2020. https://www.kff.org/coronavirus-covid-19/report/kff-covid-19-vaccine-monitor-december-2020/.

- Heller, Jean. "The Legacy of Tuskegee." *St. Petersburg Times,* July 20, 1997. Archived from the original on October 1, 2005.

- HPV Information Center. *Mongolia: Human Papillomavirus and Related Cancers, Fact Sheet 2018.* 2019. https://hpvcentre.net/statistics/reports/MNG_FS.pdf.

- Jones, James H. *Bad Blood: The Tuskegee Syphilis Experiment.* New York: The Free Press, 1981.

- Katz, Ralph V., Lee B. Green, Nancy R. Kressin, S. Stephen Kegeles, Min Qi Wang, Sherman A. James, Stephanie L. Russell, Cristina Claudio, Jan M. McCallum "The Legacy of the Tuskegee Syphilis Study: Assessing its Impact on Willingness to Participate in Biomedical Studies." *Journal of Health Care for the Poor and Underserved* 19, no. 4 (2018): 1168–1180. doi:10.1353/hpu.0.0067.

- Magner, Lois N. and Oliver Kim. *A History of Medicine.* Boca Raton: Taylor & Francis Group, 2018.

- Mayo Clinic. "Syphilis." Accessed May 10, 2021. https://www.mayoclinic.org/diseases-conditions/syphilis/symptoms-causes/syc-20351756.

- Reverby, Susan. *Examining Tuskegee: The Infamous Syphilis Study and its Legacy.* Chapel Hill: The University of North Carolina Press, 2009.

- Thomas, Stephen B. & Sandra Crouse Quinn. "Light on the Shadow of the Syphilis Study at Tuskegee." *Health Promotion Practice* 1, no. 3 (2000): 234-7. doi:10.1177/152483990000100306.

- Vonderlehr, R.A., T. Clark, O.C. Wenger, J.R. Heller. "Untreated Syphilis in the Male Negro." *Journal of Venereal Disease Information* 17 (1936): 260-265.

- Williams, K. J. "The Introduction of 'Chemotherapy' Using Arsphenamine - The First Magic Bullet." *Journal of the Royal Society of Medicine* 102, no. 8 (2009): 343–348. https://doi.org/10.1258/jrsm.2009.09k036.

CHAPTER 5: THE SAFFRON GODDESS

- Balasundaram, Prerna. "Global Maternal Healthcare: A Study in Cultural Competency." April 8, 2019. In *Matters of State*. Podcast, MP3 Audio. http://www.mattersofstate.org/global-maternal-healthcare-a-study-in-cultural-competency/.

- Banerjee, Poulomi. "Voices in Their Heads: How India Deals with Mental Disorders." *Hindustan Times*, July 12, 2015. www.hindustantimes.com/health-and-fitness/voices-in-their-heads-how-india-deals-with-mental-disorders/story-a64Jhyk4072k6SV1Ke7WdJ.html.

- Belli, Brita. "Ancient Chinese Medicine Unlocks New Possibilities for Cancer Treatment." Yale School of Medicine. press release, March 13, 2020. Yale. website. https://medicine.yale.edu/news-article/23149/.

- Chadda, R. K., & K.S. Deb (2013). "Indian Family Systems, Collectivistic Society and Psychotherapy." *Indian Journal of Psychiatry* 55, no. 2 (2013): S299–S309. http://doi.org/10.4103/0019-5545.105555.

- Farnsworth, Norman A. and Djaja Doel Soejarto. "Potential Consequence of Plant Extinction in the United States on the Current and Future Availability of Prescription Drugs." *Economic Botany* 39, no. 3 (1985): 231-240. https://doi.org/10.1007/BF02858792.

- Garg, Ishan. "Mental Health Disorder: The Demon That Keeps on Taking." *ThePost24,* June 2, 2017. https://thepost24.com/mental-health-disorder-demon-keeps-taking/.

- Gopalkrishnan, Narayan, and Hurriyet Babacan. "Cultural Diversity and Mental Health."*Australasian Psychiatry* 23, no. 6 (2015): 6-8. doi: 10.1177/1039856215609769.

- Iyer, Malathy. "7.5% Indians Suffer from Mental Disorders: WHO Report." *The Times of India*, February 25, 2017. https://timesofindia.indiatimes.com/india/7-5-indians-suffer-from-mental-disorders-who-report/articleshow/57344807.cms.

- Kennedy, Miranda. "India's Mentally Ill Turn To Faith, Not Medicine." *NPR*, August 10, 2010. https://www.npr.org/templates/story/story.php?storyId=126143778.

- Kumar, Anant. "Mental Health Services in Rural India: Challenges and Prospects." *Health* 3, no. 12 (2011): 757-761. doi:10.4236/health.2011.312126.

- Luhrmann, Tanya M., R. Padmavati, Hema Tharoor, and Akwasi Osei. "Hearing Voices in Different Cultures: A Social Kindling Hypothesis." *Topics in Cognitive Science* 7, no. 4 (2015): 646–663. doi:10.1111/tops.12158.

- Miles, Steven H. *The Hippocratic Oath and the Ethics of Medicine.* New York: Oxford University Press, 2004.

- Murthy, Srinivasa R. "Human Resources for Mental Health Care in India – Challenges and Opportunities." *Indian Journal of Psychiatry* 46, no. 4 (2004): 361-366.

- Singh, Akashdeep. "Treatment of Mental Illness in India." *CMAJ : Canadian Medical Association Journal* 176, no. 13 (2007): 1862. doi:10.1503/cmaj.1070045.

- *TEDx.* "Fayth Parks: How Culture Connects to Healing and Recovery." March 16, 2015. Video, 2:20. https://www.youtube.com/watch?v=q9Tkb879dsY.

- UW Medicine Department of Bioethics and Humanities. "Complementary Medicine." Accessed October 16, 2021. https://depts.washington.edu/bhdept/ethics-medicine/bioethics-topics/detail/57.

- Vastag, Brian. "Garlic and HIV Medication." *JAMA* 287, no. 3 (2002). doi:10.1001/jama.287.3.308-JHA10014-2-1.

- World Health Organization. *Mental Health Atlas: India.* 2011. https://www.who.int/mental_health/evidence/atlas/profiles/ind_mh_profile.pdf?ua=1.

- World Health Organization. *Mental Health Atlas: United States of America.* 2011. https://www.who.int/mental_health/evidence/atlas/profiles/usa_mh_profile.pdf?ua=1&ua=1.

CHAPTER 6: THE SAFFRON GODDESS

- Rittenhouse, Madison. "Mexican Culture: Cold and Flu Cures." *Pimsleur* (blog). September 30, 2019. https://blog.pimsleur.com/2019/09/30/mexican-cold-flu-cures/.

- Sini, Rozina. "Publisher Apologises for 'Racist' Text in Medical Book." *BBC News,* October 20, 2017. https://www.bbc.com/news/blogs-trending-41692593.

- Tervalon, Melanie and Jann-Murray Garcia. "Cultural Humility versus Cultural Competency: A Critical Distinction in Defining Physician Training Outcomes in Multicultural Education." *Journal of Health Care for the Poor and Underserved* 9, no. 2 (1998): 117-125. doi:10.1353/hpu.2010.0233.

CHAPTER 7: THE ART OF TEACHING

- Arlinghaus, Katherine R. and Craig A Johnston. "Advocating for Behavior Change With Education." *American Journal of Lifestyle Medicine* 12, no. 2 (2017): 113-116. doi:10.1177/1559827617745479.

- Bandlamudi, Adhiti. "'Cultural Brokers for Our Families': Young Vietnamese Americans Fight Online Misinformation for the Community." *KQED*, May 12, 2021. https://www.kqed.org/news/11872941/cultural-brokers-for-our-families-young-vietnamese-americans-fight-online-misinformation-for-the-community.

- Borofsky, Amelia Rachel Hokule'a. "In Some Cultures, a Role for Shame in Addressing Obesity?" *The Atlantic,* February 15, 2013. https://www.theatlantic.com/health/archive/2013/02/in-some-cultures-a-role-for-shame-in-addressing-obesity/272999/.

- "COVID-19 Vaccination Drive 2021 in Raleigh, NC." *BAPS Charities,* April 27, 2021. https://www.bapscharities.org/usa/raleigh/news/covid19-vaccinationdrive2021-12/.

- Henderson, Emily. "Study Sheds Light on the Impact of COVID-19 on Ethnocultural Communities." *News-Medical,* August 9, 2021. https://www.news-medical.net/news/20210809/Study-sheds-light-on-the-impact-of-COVID-19-on-ethnocultural-communities.aspx.

- Hoffman, Jan. "Clergy Preach Faith in the Covid Vaccine to Doubters." *New York Times*, March 14, 2021. https://www.nytimes.com/2021/03/14/health/clergy-covid-vaccine.html.

- Hoffman, Jan. "Minority Pastors Preach for the Covid Vaccine." *Arkansas Times,* March 20, 2021. https://www.arkansasonline.com/news/2021/mar/20/minority-pastors-preach-for-the-covid-vaccine/.

- Jaisinghani, Priya, et al. "COVID-19 Vaccination Failure Week 2 and Week 3 Updates." https://miro.com/app/board/o9J_lWH7U4s=/.

- Mayerle, Jennifer. "'Cultural Brokers' Work To Bridge Gaps In Equitable Vaccine Distribution." *CBS Minnesota,* March 25, 2021. https://minnesota.cbslocal.com/2021/03/25/cultural-brokers-work-to-bridge-gaps-in-equitable-vaccine-distribution/.

- NRC-RIM (National Resource Center for Refugees, Immigrants, and Migrants). *COVID Champions: Trusted Faith Leaders.* 2021. https://nrcrim.org/covid-champions-trusted-faith-leaders.

- Raynor, T., A Blenkinsopp, P Knapp, et al. "A Systematic Review of Quantitative and Qualitative Research on the Role and Effectiveness of Written Information Available to Patients About Individual Medicines." *Health Technology Assessment* 11, no. 1 (2007): 1-160. https://doi.org/10.3310/hta11050.

- Sesin, Carmen. "Latino Churches Push Covid Vaccine Enrollment, but Some Spread Misinformation." *NBC News,* March 9, 2021. https://www.nbcnews.com/news/latino/latino-churches-push-covid-vaccine-enrollment-spread-misinformation-rcna370.

- Wall, Alix. "Survivor, Antiques Dealer Tamara Katz 90." *The Jewish News of Northern California*, December 3, 2004.

- Weise, Elizabeth. "Clarity for Catholics: It's OK to Get Johnson & Johnson COVID-19 Vaccine – If It's the Only One Available." *USA Today*, March 17, 2021. https://www.usatoday.com/story/news/health/2021/03/17/johnson-johnson-covid-19-vaccine-catholics-vatican-coronavirus/4681486001/.

CHAPTER 8: THE CONSTANT OF CHANGE

- Boas, Franz. *Race, Language, and Culture.* New York: Macmillan, 1888.

- IDLO (International Development Law Organization). *Mongolia: Hand in Hand Against Domestic Violence.* 2016. https://www.idlo.int/fr/news/highlights/mongolia-hand-hand-against-domestic-violence

- *TEDx.* "Pellegrino Riccardi: Cross Cultural Communication." October 21, 2014. Video, 0:29. https://www.youtube.com/watch?v=YMyofREc5Jk.

CHAPTER 9: BALANCING ACT

- Cantor, Joel C. and Dawne M. Mouzon. "Are Hispanic, Black, and Asian Physicians Truly Less Burned Out Than White Physicians? Individual and Institutional Considerations." *JAMA Network Open* 3, no. 8 (August 2020) doi:10.1001/jamanetworkopen.2020.13099.

- Garcia, Luis C., Tait D. Shanafelt, Colin P. West, et al. "Burnout, Depression, Career Satisfaction, and Work-Life Integration by Physician Race/Ethnicity." *JAMA Network Open* 3, no. 8 (August 2020) doi:10.1001/jamanetworkopen.2020.12762.

- Narayana, Sirisha. "A Great Many Things More." Feb. 6, 2018. In *The Nocturnists*. Produced by Emily Silverman. Podcast, MP3 Audio. https://thenocturnists.com/season1/2018/5/8/2-a-great-many-things-more.

CHAPTER 10: CROSSING CIRCLES

- Kumar, Ashwani. "Hindu Doctor, Raised in Dubai, Recites Kalima Shahada for Dying Covid Patient." *Khaleej Times,* May 21, 2021. https://www.khaleejtimes.com/coronavirus-pandemic/hindu-doctor-raised-in-dubai-recites-kalima-shahada-for-dying-covid-patient.

- Mirror Now Digital. "'A Humane Act'! Hindu Doctor Reels Off Islamic Prayer in Dying Muslim COVID-19 Patient's Ears in Kerala." *Mirror Now News,* May 21, 2021. https://www.timesnownews.com/mirror-now/in-focus/article/a-humane-act-hindu-doctor-reels-off-islamic-prayer-in-dying-muslim-covid-19-patient-s-ears-in-kerala/759793.

- Panchap, Latha. "Not Cut Out For This." Nov. 17, 2020. In *The Nocturnists.* Produced by Emily Silverman. Podcast, MP3 Audio. https://thenocturnists.com/season-3/2020/11/17/s3-ep8-not-cut-out-for-this.

- Statista. *Amount of Time U.S. Primary Care Physicians Spent with Each Patient as of 2018.* 2019. https://www.statista.com/statistics/250219/us-physicians-opinion-about-their-compensation/.

- White-Hammond, Gloria. "African-American Spirituality, Illness, and the COVID-19 Crisis." Sept. 18, 2020. In *Duke Theology, Medicine, and Culture Initiative.* Produced by Duke Divinity School. Podcast, MP3 Audio. https://soundcloud.com/duketmc/rev-gloria-white-hammond-md-african-american-spirituality-illness-and-the-covid-19-crisis.